DIVORCE YOUR DIET

HOLLAN GOEWEY

DIVORCE YOUR DIET

AND LIVE HEALTHILY EVER AFTER

Urano
publishing

Argentina - Chile - Colombia - Spain
USA - Mexico - Peru - Uruguay

© 2024 *by* Hollan Goewey

© 2024 by Urano Publishing, an imprint of Urano World USA, Inc

8871 SW 129th Terrace Miami FL 33176 USA

Urano
publishing

Cover art and design by Sandra de Waard

Cover copyright © Urano Publishing, an imprint of Urano World USA, Inc

The first edition of this book was published in February 2024

ISBN: 978-1-953027-33-7

E-ISBN: 978-1-953027-35-1

Printed in Colombia

Library of Cataloging-in-Publication Data

Goewey, Hollan

1. Health & Wellness   2. Nutrition

Divorce Your Diet

TABLE OF CONTENTS

As a lifelong vegetarian and proponent of the healing power of food, I know firsthand the impact that plant-based foods and natural medicines can have on the body. My parents were my guiding light in this journey, introducing me to the wonders of wheatgrass, tofu, chia seeds, and fermented foods at a young age.

It was in the early 90s, when I was just 15 years old, that my parents brought Kombucha into our household. At first, the unusual taste and smell of the fermented tea turned me off, but I quickly changed my mind when I saw the positive impact it had on my family, particularly my mother during her battle with breast cancer.

I began brewing my own Kombucha with the intention of sharing its benefits with as many people as possible. Every batch I brew is a living reminder of this purpose, to improve people's lives and make the world a better place. As the founder and CEO of GT's Living Foods, my North star is to make the best product possible and to help people live better lives through health and wellness.

That's why I was thrilled to meet Hollan, a like-minded soul who believes in the power of healthy and delicious food. As a chef on Kauai, Hollan has a unique talent for taking traditional foods and giving them a healthy twist. From spice-rubbed jackfruit tacos to smoked eggplant meatballs, her dishes are a testament to the delicious possibilities of plant-based eating.

Hollan also shares my passion for fermented foods and uses my products to make her dishes even healthier. From using our Synergy Gingerade Kombucha in dressings to adding a healthy spin to spinach dip with Cocoyo, our raw young coconut yogurt,

Hollan is a master at incorporating health into the foods you already love.

That's why I'm excited to write the foreword for this book, which delves into the world of replacing traditional foods with healthier options. The best way to achieve optimal health is by replacing foods that detract from our well-being with ones that nourish and sustain us. This book is the guide to help you on that journey.

Cheers to your health,

GT Dave
Founder and CEO of GT's Living Foods

WHO IS HOLLAN?

Most likely you don't know me, so let me introduce myself. A search online of my bio states, "Hollan Goewey is a Cordon Bleu-trained chef, health advocate, former restaurant owner, and mom of three. She has been vegan for 15 years, and she loves creating new plant-based recipes to get you to eat healthier without realizing it. True to her beach-inspired lifestyle, Hollan lives on the beautiful garden isle of Kauai and enjoys spending time in the kitchen, and in the rejuvenating waters of the Pacific Ocean, with family and friends."

Living on the Hawaiian island of Kauai makes me feel like one of the Lost Boys living in Neverland. I am always exploring and enjoying nature, practicing headstands in the sand, and watching chickens and birds run through my yard. Even though it sometimes feels like Peter Pan's home, let's be real, this isn't Neverland. No place is perfect, no life is perfect. But we can try to make our lives BETTER. When I began to change how I looked at food as a way to health, I also found vitality and energy, which made me a more positive human. In one sense, wherever you go, there you are. Both in a literal and metaphorical sense. The statement "we are what we eat" is true. I have found that this vitality and positivity follow me wherever I go and has flourished over the years. Are there times that I fall out of this?

Absolutely, but I know what I can do to help bring myself back to this healthy space. My goal became to help others learn this about themselves too. I am not a doctor, but I learned what worked for me, and have helped others learn what works for them. Hopefully, through reading this book, you are able to learn and accept what works for you.

I grew up in the San Francisco Bay Area, and loved the variety of foods I had all around me. One of six kids, meals at my house were always about feeding the masses as easily as you could. Growing up a vegetarian by choice in a meat-centered household, my mom always made me a veggie version of whatever she concocted. My grandmother always entertained in style, and signed me up for etiquette classes. Now I find my style is somewhere in between the two. As a teenager I began adding meat to my diet in order to not stand out or be perceived as difficult. I have always loved food and it was not until I started traveling in my teens that I realized how special and diverse the food scene in San Francisco is.

During a brief modeling career, I used food to keep my body at a certain weight (this was during 90s waif craze). From there, my love affair with food was an on again/off again fling. Once I became pregnant, this statement became even more true. It moved my love of food up on the scale. After they were born, I restricted what I ate to lose weight.

I realized I was pregnant when one day a friend of mine commented how much I had been loving food recently. I hadn't made the connection of how much or what I was eating, to the changes happening in my body. After my son was born, I attempted to be what I thought was the perfect stay at home mom. I would plan and cook 3-course meals every night. Even though it could be stressful, I learned that I actually loved planning, cooking, and entertaining. I took a leap, and, with a toddler in tow, decided to put myself through culinary school, specializing in pastries at Cordon Bleu in San Francisco. When I was in culinary school, I had another love affair with food, and then restricted to lose the weight I had gained eating my way through it.

After graduating and having my second child, I chose restaurant jobs that were front of house. Being a server often meant shorter hours and better pay than kitchen jobs. I worked in hotels and dining for 10 years and my obsession with food, entertaining, and catering grew. I would always be sneaking off to the kitchens to peek at the day's menu and see the chefs at work. From there, I started working in the catering business, planning events, serving, and managing restaurants and hotels.

With dreams of living in Hawaii, I packed up my family and we made the move across the Pacific. While there, I had my third child. The pregnancy was harder than the others and I was diagnosed with gestational diabetes. After she was born, it was harder to lose the pregnancy weight. I was also beginning to have some autoimmune symptoms that were plaguing my life. After some research, and many different yo-yo diets, I decided to try eating vegan. This was a new adventure and I was able to use the culinary skills I had learned in school with new ingredients to create scrumptiously delicious vegan food. My health drastically changed. Eating vegan, and being vegan, changed my life. I became obsessed. Once I had children and started learning about nutrition, I wanted more for them than what I had, more knowledge and more health.

While working in restaurants and hotels, I decided to try my luck and applied to be a contestant on the popular American game show, *Wheel of Fortune*! My then husband and I were chosen to participate, and after what seemed like fate pushing us along, we won! I decided to use our Wheel of Fortune winnings to purchase a small cafe. Owning the restaurant gave me the time I needed to perfect my art, which is homestyle vegan cooking. All of these recipes have been tested by my family, my kids, and the thousands of customers who walked through our doors.

Years later, I sold the restaurant and began writing books. My first book, a lifestyle cookbook, called *Good Food Gratitude*, came out in 2019. These are some of the reasons why I can give qualified opinions on this subject, but the main reason is really because I have been dieting in some shape or form since realizing that society judges you based on how you look. Every magazine cover seemed to validate this belief. I found my health through going vegan, but continued to diet when I was feeling great. I have tried calorie counting, water fasting, raw veganism, intermittent fasting, juicing, Paleo, and Keto. Guess what I learned? FUCK DIETING. It doesn't work in the long run, it doesn't lead you to health, and that is why I am writing this book.

I am lucky enough that I am able to visit friends and family all over the world. My travels are always focused on what I love—sharing my recipes, learning new recipes, exploring flavors, and experiencing other cultures. I love going out into the world, meeting new people, and trying their delicious dishes. It's amazing to me how long traditions stick around. I guess that's why they call it tradition? Sometimes you can even feel love and emotion through someone cooking food for you. I love to challenge myself to deconstruct and recreate my favorite flavors with a vegan spin. I want to show people that you can still honor our world's traditions, even when altering aspects of our meals by making them healthier.

I'm just a normal girl, well, I guess I should say woman, who is looking for vitality in life. I want to tend to my temple, but I also want to enjoy life and not feel restricted on things I want. We all know the difference between feeling good and not good, or healthy and not healthy. I am not training for a triathlon. I will never run a marathon. Most of the time I have to talk myself into working out because my brain tends to be a bit lazy. I want to take short cuts, like saying that I'm always busy and make excuses for not doing it. But I want to choose life, so I know I am up against a lazy, excuse-making part of myself every day. I choose to take care of myself and my food choices, and move my body as it was meant to, with either a walk, yoga, or a workout. This book is the culmination of my life and relationship with food and what I found to be the balance to stay somewhere in the middle and feel like you're in control. I'm not here to get you into the best shape of your life, unless that's what you want. I'm here to teach you what I've learned so that you can have a relationship with healthy food. **Toxic is so out. Self-respect is so in.**

XO,
Hollan

INTRODUCTION

Divorce your Diet. Break up with your beliefs. Health is like a never-ending puzzle where you are trying to simply feed a body that is rather complex. There are so many pieces to the puzzle, most people don't know where to start. A lot of people treat the puzzle pieces without realizing that you can't have health without the puzzle being put together. There is no instruction book or way to know how you are doing, except by checking in with how you feel. There are various alarms that our body sets off, but we don't always know how to read them. There is no manual for the natural alarms your body is constantly sending you. Considering there are 80,000 body processes happening at once, like digesting food and processing nutrients, it is hard to differentiate or guess what is causing your symptoms. Those symptoms can feel like bloating, constipation, lack of energy, depression, and long-term inflammatory pain. The symptoms don't look the same for everyone. If we ignore the symptoms they can pile up and cause more damage to our bodies. Eating is a mindful practice we all do, like breathing, but never really talk about it or really learn about it. I mean it is rarely mentioned that FOOD is the cornerstone to health. Even when we get blood work done, we don't get a full picture of our health.

It's hard to figure out how to get to health from the snapshot that Western medicine gives us. We all know someone perceived as healthy who has had a disease or someone (maybe even yourself!) that has an autoimmune disease and can't keep it under control. The goal is to start to see it as simple, not science, when it comes to our bodies. It becomes simple when you know to check in with yourself and see how many of the foods we eat put us into an autoimmune response. Many people believe that there is a right way to eat. They sell you their diet, one they probably don't follow themselves, that in the short term will work, but leads you to a dead end where you find yourself more confused about how to find health.

Perhaps you've dieted and found a diet that worked for you, but you fell off and you think that if you just ate that way again you would have the body and health you want. Maybe it's keto, paleo, raw vegan, Atkins, or whatever the latest craze is. I am sorry to say that this isn't true, there is no right diet for everyone. Humans have vast needs, and many of them aren't being met because we aren't eating a diet that is high in actual nutrition. However, our bodies are also amazing in that they store many nutrients, so we don't actually need to get all of our nutritional needs met daily. Vitamin and protein shake sellers and diet slingers make us think we need them too. They tell us that their path is the right one, while totally ignoring that humans have diverse nutritional needs, which can change throughout their lives. For example, humans generally don't drink breast milk past early childhood, because we don't need it anymore, and we get those nutrients from whole foods. To make things more complicated, the body isn't in optimal health when it is unable to access quality nutrients stored in its system, so we start to have other health issues. There is such a thing as too much nutrition. When your body has enough stored and you continuously give it more, your body has to work harder to remove and use those nutrients.

This brings me to my next point. There is no right way to eat all the time. It's about divorcing yourself from someone else's plan and learning about food and your body's needs. It's as simple as replacing the ingredients in the food that you eat. When I first started using food to try to come to health, I started to see that there wasn't one way to eat. I did all types of diets and started to see that I was stuck in a loop of thinking there could be better diets and that I could feel better, both mentally and physically. But nope, I was chasing health and weight loss, instead of being present in my body and my body's needs.

All diets work at first, because we become conscious of what we are putting into our bodies. We aren't on auto pilot. We are planning. We also eat way less or simpler on any diet. Our bodies require 6 nutrients: **vitamins, minerals, protein, fats, water, and carbohydrates** to convert food into nutrition.

Nutrition to me is trying to use food or supplements to have my body be in homeostasis, where it is working for me. Based on what I was eating, I was able to help myself. Changing what I ate helped me to have a healthier future. Food matters. Food is supposed to be energy and body-building. In the past we relied on our senses to help us hunt and gather food. It took more than going to the market to get our food, and our senses, like taste and smell, would help us sniff it out and determine if it was safe or not. We now use these senses to get pleasure from food. We use it to please the senses. Most of the time we don't think about its implications once it's in the body. This in turn has us completely ignoring the fact that food is energy.

When I started changing my health, I went vegan and used my culinary skills to change all my favorite foods into a vegan version. When I went on someone else's diet, it worked for a little bit, but then I missed my foods and would fall back into my old diet. This left me in a loop of indulgence, then deprivation, then indulgence again, all while wreaking havoc on my system. I started working with clients and they were the same. They would all say, "if I could just follow that one diet where I saw change, I would find my health and where I want my body to be." This isn't true though. Because no one diet is for all of us, all of the time, which is why there is such an abundance of food throughout different seasons, with a diversity of vitamins, minerals, carbs, fats, and proteins. We are supposed to get our nutrients from the wide variety of nutrition that different foods offer.

Throughout this journey you will be learning about your body, how to break up with old beliefs about food, how to create the foods you love with better ingredients, how to listen to your body when it inevitably falls in and out of health, and how to take care of yourself physically and mentally when it does. Even though it may sound like a lot, I'm going to show you how simple it can be! You can have your cake and eat it too. Believe me, as someone who went to pastry school for her love of sweets, divorcing your diet can taste better than you would ever believe.

You may learn or read some things you don't want to hear, but ignorance on taking care of yourself is not bliss for your body. Education is the key to learning how to tend to your temple. Be open.

I am going to teach you the basics of food as I know it. I am a chef, not a nutritionist. We are learning more and more about food and what they taught 30 years ago has changed, and it will change in 30 more years. As we learn, we evolve.

Chapter 1

DIVORCE YOUR DIET

Then vs. Now, What Divorcing My Diet Has Given Me

Y ou are in a toxic relationship with ingredients. It's not you, it's them. Both the ingredients and the companies making your ingredients. All you have to do is leave them to find something healthier that works for YOU. It's hard for me to state my case considering that I am not a scientist, a doctor, or a nutritionist. However, I am a chef, a mom, a writer, and, for most of my life, I have battled with my weight or the thought that being skinnier meant being healthier and happier.

In my teens, I was modeling during the waif craze, and I was miserable as I tried to keep my weight at 105 pounds. When I became pregnant with my third baby, my weight was at an all-time high for me, 180 pounds. I was diagnosed with gestational diabetes, which led me to more diets, like eating paleo and Atkins. I was raised on the "standard American diet," aka SAD. My favorite foods were processed and full of sugar and chemicals. While on meat-heavy diets, I cut out carbs, and ate more meat than vegetables. While I found I could alleviate some of my symptoms for a short time, throughout this ordeal I never found health.

The weight was still there, the symptoms were still there, and I was not getting healthier or feeling better. It wasn't just the weight that was affecting me, I was also suffering from an auto-immune disease. I had surgery twice for endometriosis and I had kidney stones. The icing on the cake was that, at 30, I lost my energy and vitality and couldn't get the weight off from my third pregnancy. It was not only affecting my perception of myself but my physical health as well.

I knew something had to change in me. My biggest obstacle was my love of food, like real true love. I love making it, I love eating it, I love creating new recipes, I just love it. I went to culinary school because of my love of food, so how could the things I'd fallen in love with be part of what was hurting me?

I mean I ate veggies daily, and I promised myself I would work out more. Working out gave me a little bump of energy and I got more in shape while staying overweight. My symptoms continued. In 2007, I read a book that changed my life, *Skinny Bitch* by Rory Freedman and Kim Barnounin. I was vegan within a week of reading it.

Simply stated, a person who is vegan does not eat any products made from or with animal products—this includes meat, cheese, milk from animals, eggs, and honey. There are many facets to veganism, and, for some, that may include not using any products made from animals, such as leather or beeswax.

I know that this way of eating sounds so boring to anyone who doesn't know a lot about plant foods. There are so many amazing options out there. You can find replacements for everything. This book is all about changing your life by changing your habits. It won't always be easy, but the outcome will absolutely be worth it.

Over the subsequent weeks, months, and years, I changed my life with the power of food. I changed my cooking style to one based on fruits, vegetables, and plant-based products. For the first time in my life I felt in control of my health. Rather quickly, I was able to reverse my ailments, get my vitality back, lose the weight, and build a better relationship with my body.

This was in 2007 and there were very few choices on the market in terms of vegan food, and even fewer vegan restaurants. I took my culinary education and started crafting yummy vegan recipes of my favorite meals with healthier ingredients. I was eating the food I loved, but in a different way. Most importantly to me, I was losing weight, and feeling better. I was in control of my health and the way I felt. I divorced my old way of eating and got into a healthy relationship with food. Does this mean that I'm perfect and have it all figured out? Absolutely not! There are times where I feel my health plateau, but through a more intuitive approach to the foods I eat I am always able to find a healthy balance and get back to vitality.

This is why you need to divorce your diet and just eat what you love, but healthier.

I still have to pay attention to my health, but I have built a stronger relationship with my body. I now have an understanding of what I need and what helps me feel my absolute best. I also have an understanding of what foods bring me out of health and make me feel like shit. By no means am I saying that you, yes you, the person reading this right now, needs to be a vegan. There are so many things within the vegan diet that I think can help you. I want to help you divorce your diet and create a lifestyle where you include more fruits, vegetables, and plant-based foods daily.

I know that veganism, and vegans, can have a bad reputation. I'd like to shed some light on this. People go vegan for three reasons.

1. For their love of animals.
2. For their health.
3. For the planet and the environment.

Although eating shouldn't be political, it is. I tend to fall under category number 2, and 1 and 3 are bonuses to me. I have found that people who became vegan because of categories 1 and 3 are so passionate about veganism that they close people off from wanting to eat vegan at all. I want to clarify that a lot of what we face in humanity and on our planet is very real. Compassion is important. I'm asking you to be open. Try it. See if you can change any preconceived notions you might have. If you have some heated feelings towards veganism or vegans, try changing your mindset.

You are what you eat. It's time to elaborate on this. You are *everything* you ingest. From the time you wake up in the morning, until you go to bed at night, you truly are what you eat. Food sets your mood, food sets your energy level, food sets your digestion. Food literally is your fuel. So why don't we pay more attention to what we eat and put in our bodies? One reason is because we are confused. Every day we are given contradictory information. We live in a world of diet culture that uses the fact we haven't been food educated against us. Another reason is medical professionals only receive minimal education on food and nutrition. (Minor) Very often, the prescriptions from our doctors are pills to help mask our symptoms instead of being informed about the food we eat. I am not putting down modern medicine, I am merely pointing out that, when it comes to our health, it is more often sick care than health care. Why not take care of ourselves and use food as prevention?

I am all about antibiotics or medicine that helps when you need it, but a lot of diseases or autoimmune disorders are caused by your diet, and a pill can't change that or your immunity.

If you Google "What is the definition of food?", this is what you'll see:

Food, substance consisting essentially of protein, carbohydrate, fat, and other nutrients used in the body of an organism to sustain growth and vital processes and to furnish energy. The absorption and utilization of food by the body is fundamental to nutrition and is facilitated by digestion.

This definition doesn't really tell you what food is or, more importantly, how your body uses it. One point that stands out to me in this simple definition is that food should give you nutrition, it should support vital processes in your body, like brain function, energy, and digestion.

Most people think of food as pleasure. That food is here to tickle your taste buds—which is true—but it needs to be relative to the way we use those nutrients. In our modern culture, that burger may be what you're craving and it may hit the spot, but most likely it will drain your energy instead of providing it for you. If you were on a long walk and hadn't eaten for days and came across a watermelon field, it would probably taste amazing and give you energy. It is confusing that certain foods taste good to us, but don't provide nutrition or energy. Fuck that. I want my cake and to eat it too.

Food can taste good and help us be our best selves. Our society loves to promote diet culture. We have become addicted to indulging in all these foods, and then attempt to repair ourselves, by restricting and dieting. We follow this cycle, but never gain an appreciation for quality foods and a better understanding of nutrition.

Now that we have a better understanding of food as energy (the substances we need to provide us the energy we burn throughout the day) let's talk about your new ex, diets and diet culture.

There are a few definitions for the word diet (di·et |dīət | Noun) including, but not limited to:

1. The kinds of food that a person, animal, or community habitually eats: *a vegetarian diet | a specialist in diet.*

   • a regular occupation or series of activities in which one participates: *a healthy diet of classical music.*

2. A special course of food to which one restricts oneself, either to lose weight or for medical reasons: *I'm going on a diet.*

   • *[as modifier]* (of food or drink) with reduced fat or sugar content: *diet soft drinks.*

Most of us find ourselves using the latter definition. Notice the word RESTRICT. So many diets that we try either for weight loss, or to build health and muscle, or to feel better than we do, often focuses on this word, restriction. Diets often either require you to restrict what you eat, or how much or when you eat. A lot of times, the advice is to eat smaller amounts or less calories while completely ignoring the quality of food, which is what matters, or to shorten the hours in the day in which you eat. Often times we are told that quantity of food = health, when in reality quality of food = health.

Once you dive in and learn about high-quality foods and ingredients, you'll see that you don't have to restrict what you eat. You just need fewer and better ingredients, like organic, simple foods. This is the whole point of divorcing your diet—just like the end of a relationship, it's not about them, it's about you! How can you make a lifestyle change for the better? Better for you, better for animals, better for the planet. Divorcing your diet isn't about restriction and getting rid of the foods that are bad for you. It's about a shift and replacing those foods with ones that will love you more than your ex. Doesn't that sound amazing?

A lot of times these restrictive diets work for us for a couple of months, and then we tend to plateau. Either from sabotaging ourselves (I'll just eat that one cookie which quickly turns into 10) or from having set unrealistic habits, like fasting or restricting before a busy day at work and running out of energy before 10 AM. Divorcing your diet frees you from the yo-yo and quick gains and losses of dieting. It helps you to feel better about the choices you make, and gives you the ability to forgive yourself when you make unhealthy choices, which we all (yes, even me!) sometimes make.

Besides easing yourself from the horrible reality of restriction, divorcing your diet is also about learning about yourself. What foods make you feel good and provide you the energy you need? How is the food that you're eating helping or hindering your body and your health? The goal of letting go of that nasty ex is to better understand yourself, your wants, and needs, while also helping your body in the long term.

Ultra-processed foods entered the food scene around 60 years ago. A recent study showed that more than half of the average American diet is these ultra-processed foods. (Fox) During this time, we have also seen an increase in diseases like cancer in people under 50. (Communications) Diabetes, high blood pressure, and autoimmune disorders continue to rise. It is one of those things that is so simple and obvious. Could the way we have changed our foods have a direct impact on our health? As these varieties of prepackaged foods grew, so did disease and health problems. Oftentimes the first recommendation is to take different medications, but let's take it back to Hippocrates (aka the Father of Medicine, "let food be thy medicine and medicine be the food") and remember that our first starting place to health should be our food. Fortunately for him, when Hippocrates said this, fast food and prepackaged openly modified foods weren't being advertised and thrown at him on a daily basis. It feels like it is harder than ever to break up with this industry and culture that is trying to sabotage us incessantly. I'm here to show you that it is much simpler than you think, and once you ditch crap foods that are undeserving of your time and energy you will begin to reap the benefits almost immediately. Like a bad relationship, sometimes it's hard for us to see how bad it is for us when we are in it. But, once we take a step back, after a couple of weeks we have 20/20 vision.

Here are some things for you to think about before taking this leap of faith. And it really is a leap of faith. Not belief in me, but in yourself. Divorcing your diet is about getting rid of the toxic diet culture and finding simple solutions, but it is also about starting to realize how powerful you are in your own right. There is really nothing more powerful than being able to take charge of your habits and your health.

So, before serving papers to your toxic habits, I want to know:

1. Do you eat the same foods every day?

2. Are you food educated?

3. Do you read ingredient labels on packaged foods?

4. Do you think there is one way for you to eat?

5. Do you crave your favorite meals from your childhood and beyond?

6. Do you care about conventionally grown fruits and veggies (grown with pesticides) versus organic (non-GMO and pesticide free)?

I have come to find that nothing affects our health more than our daily habits. We eat daily. Actually, we eat throughout the day. This habit, for better and worse, can impact our bodies the most. This is the habit that probably causes more disease than any other. There is a big disconnect between our need to eat, and our understanding of what foods can bring us into health.

First things first—let's talk about your body and get some basic knowledge of how the body works and what it needs. Then, we will draft those divorce papers and see why you need to break up with your diet... and lose some of those food beliefs.

Indulge and Repair or Repair and Indulge?

Many people I know live to indulge and then repair. They party all weekend, eat shit foods, and make excuses that this behavior is okay or deserving because they will be better during the week, never finding health. They believe they can make it up. I'll eat salad all week, I won't eat carbs. I'll drink smoothies.

I'm a believer that when you are eating healthy and staying healthy, the indulgence doesn't take over. If this sounds familiar you need to switch your ratios. Once you have set your daily habits, and you are taking care of yourself, you don't need to indulge as much. You will be in a state of repair and health, so the indulgence won't take over. I don't know how this works, but when you are in a healthy state, getting the nutrients you need, your cravings lessen and you feel satiated. On the flip side, if you are constantly indulging and trying to make up for it by eating healthier for a couple of days, your body never has the chance to heal itself. You trick your brain into thinking it is, but it needs more time. Think of it as a battle, the indulgence army versus the repair army. Who is the winner? Once you know who the winner is, have you helped yourself or is it taking you out of health? You know when you are feeling good and then you go out and have too many drinks on the weekend? Or maybe it's something like family has come for a visit and they spend the entire weekend eating BBQ food, cakes, and sweets, binging on decadent food. You feel the difference, you wake up feeling like shit. Can you repair the damage you've caused? Yes, you can repair THE DAMAGE, by loading up on foods you know bring you into health and help your cells to repair. The difference between indulging more or getting back into health puts your body into more damage or repair.

This can vary as we age, or as our bodies are in different seasons. These seasons are different for everyone and are based on how they treated their bodies when they were younger. For example, as we age, our organs don't process toxins as well as they used to. This could explain why our bodies have a greater reaction to anesthesia, drugs, stimulants, and threats. We feel it because our defenses don't work as well. There are ways to make our bodies work longer, better.

Humans live for the short term, and we love immediate rewards, like the foods we eat to quench a craving. But we don't think about how it will make us feel tomorrow or next week. That shit food at night that has us hungover in the morning. Like when you eat a pizza at 11 at night. Your body can't break that down while you're sleeping, your body needs to be moving to help it digest that food. We live for the short-term reward and we don't think about long-term health. How will eating this pizza affect my sleep? What will I want to eat tomorrow if I feel like crap? What if those immediate rewards make me feel like garbage?

Hollan's Goals:

Five goals for the body:

1. Feel more energy throughout the day

2. Lose 5 pounds

3. Tone up around my waistline

4. Love my body

5. Clear skin

Five goals for the mind:

1. Own my fear

2. Feel grateful

3. Meditate

4. Feel happy

5. Worry less

Now that you have written these goals, I want you to release the shame from yourself for not being where you want to be, yet. The reason you need to divorce your diet is because you went into it unconsciously. You are not born with a roadmap to your health. We go by what our parents and schools taught us, like eating everything on your plate to be excused, or having a glass of milk with each meal for the calcium. For me, I didn't regularly drink water, because it wasn't a habit in my household when I was a kid. Besides diets, most of us know very little about our body and its relationship with food.

This world is set up to put you into dis-ease, not health. It's not your fault. You have been set up to fail, because what you were sold isn't true and you are constantly being marketed to. Remember the sugar water ads from cola companies in the 90s? You had to drink soda to be cool. There were ads targeting us to drink milk because celebrities did. Even social media today is constantly advertising to us, regardless of whether the influencer selling it cares about how it affects our bodies or not. There are whole industries dedicated to making us buy their crap foods with crap ingredients.

There are also pictures of family farms on the packaging that paints a picture that isn't necessarily the case. This is hidden marketing. It's everywhere.

I was never given the tools, and through my experience, and working with the people I have met in the journey of my health, this is my brief understanding of the body and what you need in the most broken-down terms. I started to learn about the human body from the hundreds of practitioners I have seen over the last 15 years. I am surprised at how much I have learned in researching for this book that I didn't know. I hope you do too. My goal is to set you up for a life of health, both physically and mentally, with food at the forefront of your journey.

If you're still reading this it is likely because of your perceived relationship with food. You have already made the first step to divorce your diet. Yay! Let's dig deeper and learn more about you and the amazing role food can play in your health and body.

I want to talk about pain. We all try to avoid it, and we turn to its opposite—pleasure. When you start a diet, do you binge on everything you're giving up right before you begin? That's because our brains seek out pleasure to avoid pain. The pain is in making a change. It's not easy. Divorce is hard. It isn't meant to be easy, and that's what makes the change worth it. Like climbing a mountain and checking out the view from the summit. The view is more spectacular because you put in the work to climb. Making this change will be hard. You have to rely on seeing a pleasurable change in the future by giving up what you perceive as pleasure from food. Replacing ingredients at first was hard on my taste buds, and I missed the foods my body had been accustomed to. But soon I was craving the replacements. My perception of pleasure changed, and my body began to respond to it.

Goals are so important. They are how we see if the effort we are putting in is working.

Chapter 2

I WANT YOU TO LEARN YOU

How I Learned Me

Divorcing your diet is about educating yourself on your food, your body, and its wants and needs. Understanding health is not a destination, it's a journey of trying to get and stay in health. I have found that we have a very limited education on the mind, the body, its functions, and its relationship to food. It's important to learn about all of these if you want to divorce your diet. You need to learn about what your body needs and what your system does with those ingredients.

The Mind

Before you can accomplish anything, you have to deal with the trickiest part, the thing that controls all of your systems, your mind. Your brain, like your body, is trying to bring you back into a state of homeostasis (the body's state of being in balance). However, it also craves pleasure and serotonin (happy hormones), which can throw things off. The brain has an exact set of processes that control most of our bodies actions. Ultimately, the most freeing thing to realize is that the mind is controlled by you. The other you. The you that is talking to it. It listens and proceeds from there.

Don't get me wrong—there are a lot of autopilots happening in the brain. We have trained our brains to recognize these autopilots, and to not interfere. However, you are at the helm. You need to be able to tell it that you are trying a new way of living on foods that support you. Your brain doesn't care if that chocolate peanut butter cup is organic or made of whole foods, but your body does. This is the first step to divorce your diet, realizing you need to train your brain to show up for you. Instead of the negative talk, and continually telling yourself "you are so fat," or "you are sick," try telling it "you are healing." Since you are in a relationship with your mind, it is important that you are doing this for you. For your quality of life and to feel vitality.

It can be tough to hear. Doing this for you. I know one thing for sure, you have to do this for you. No one else, just you. You have to align with what you want, not with pleasing others.

I listen to a lot of self-help guidance, but this particularly resonated with me.

The inspirational speaker, Esther Hicks, once interviewed a woman in her audience. The audience member talked about something she wanted to give up for others, even though it was something she enjoyed. Esther's perfect response was that doing things for others is a slippery slope to failure. She said, "It's not your job to change so they can feel better, you can't change your behavior in enough ways to make them feel better. You lose weight, and then they want you to dress better. You then dress better and then they want you to buy a different kind of car. Then you buy that car, they want you to live in the state they live in. Then you'll move in the state they live in, then they'll want you to grow your hair out. Then they'll want you to cut it, then they'll want you to make it a different color, then they'll want you to act your age. You can't stand on your head in enough ways."

I love that phrase. "You can't stand on your head in enough ways." It's so true. If you're a people pleaser this will probably resonate with you. In order to help your brain heal your body, you will need to remind it that you are doing this for yourself and not for other people.

Before I divorced my diet, I was constantly standing on my head in too many ways. I was living my life to please others. Over many years, I have learned that getting the mind, health, and body you want is something you need to do for you. You have to jump through your own hoops, not ones that others have set up for you.

Recently I have seen a meme around that goes a little something like this:

"You can eat the kale, drink the alkaline water, take the supplements, do yoga, but if you don't deal with the shit going on in your heart and head you're still unhealthy."

"You can eat the kale, drink the alkaline water, take the supplements, do yoga, but if you don't deal with the shit going on in your heart and head you're still unhealthy."

I have to say this saying has been true for me. There were times where my body was where I wanted it, but the dialogue inside my mind was not. Even though I was technically the healthiest I had ever been, I wasn't always the happiest. It really can be a mental game.

Changing this meme to fit my life I would say:

"You eat the kale, drink the alkaline water, take the supplements, do yoga, and, because you also deal with the shit going on in your heart and your head, you're healthy."

But you need more than kale, alkaline water, and supplements.

Your body isn't doing its own thing. It's a package deal with your mind and your nutrition. Before you begin divorcing yourself from the multitude of diets, you have to shift your attitude and then ultimately your outlook will change, then your health, and then your life.

If you want to continue to expand your mind, check out some of my favorite books on mental health and self-guidance.

- *Awareness: The Perils and Opportunities of Reality* by Anthony DeMello
- *What I Know For Sure* by Oprah Winfrey
- *The End of Stress* by Don Joseph Goewey
- *How To Own Your Mind* by Napoleon Hill
- *Love Warrior* by Glennon Doyle
- *Atomic Habits* by James Clear
- *Breaking the Habit of Being Yourself* by Dr. Joe Dispenza
- *Becoming Supernatural* by Dr. Joe Dispenza
- *The Astonishing Power of Emotions* by Esther and Jerry Hicks

We are evolving human beings with physical and emotional highs and lows, with hormones that regulate us, and stress that affects us all over. We go through this as we age, and we store vitamins, minerals, and try our hardest to survive. It's not about a perfect recipe to be the best you, it's about learning that life is a recipe for changing and evolving our bodies and our minds.

Let's take a look at the word healthy. Another way to look at it would be to heal - thy [self]. Although we talk about healing a lot, what we are really talking about is health, because one can't exist without the other. At the root of the word healthy is heal— once you are healthy, you can heal thyself. Your mind is the first place to start. Can you make this shift and change for you? When I am in health, I make choices that support my body, and when I'm out of health, I make choices that keep me out of health. I tell myself "I can have one more cookie—it won't hurt." A healthy mind says, "I had the one cookie, I'm good, I don't need the other one." When I'm eating healthily, I also tend to think more naturally about the effect that foods will have on my body. When I feel good, I don't want to feel like shit—I try to maintain the good feeling. When I'm eating foods that don't support me (highly processed, low-to-zero nutritional value), it's like my body craves more of it, and wants to feel like shit. The only one dictating to your mind (and then your body) is YOU.

The Body

Our bodies have a whole process with food and it is complicated. There is so much happening inside of our digestive systems that we don't even realize. This system is used to process, utilize, and dispose of all the nutrients from the food we eat. It also delivers these nutrients to our cells to protect our bodies. When we eat foods that our bodies don't recognize, or know what to do with, the system protects us from those chemicals, or unknown things that enter our cells.

Here is the easiest, most digestible way to give you a crash course on what happens in your body as it processes food. It is important for us to have a snapshot of what is happening in our bodies every time we eat. The more we know, the more we want to help these systems run smoothly.

Let's talk about how food is converted into energy. This may seem boring, or even too technical, but it is important to understand how our bodies break down and digest food and nutrients.

Step 1: We eat food, and it is first broken down by our teeth and the enzymes in our saliva.

Step 2: The food moves down our esophagus and gastrointestinal tract (GI for short) tube, it ends up in the stomach, where it is digested even more and the stomach acid kills the bacteria and germs. It also produces an enzyme that breaks down proteins.

WOW—our bodies really work.

Step 3: Your stomach breaks the food down into even smaller pieces to be processed. It travels through the duodenum where more digestion and nutrient absorption occurs.

Step 4: Once in the small intestine, food is hit by different chemicals for specific components of the food ingested. Proteins, lipids (fat), and carbs (sugar) are digested by enzymes that come from the pancreas. A tube connects the pancreas to the duodenum and all the enzymes travel to the duodenum when food is in the system. A different tube connects the duodenum to the liver and gallbladder. This tube sends bile, made by the liver and stored in the gallbladder, to the food in the intestine. Bile is needed to finish the complete digestion of fat and fat-soluble vitamins A, D, E, and K.

Step 5: After the sugar (carbs) we ingest are mostly broken down by enzymes from the pancreas, the cells that line the small intestine use their enzymes to completely digest the sugars. Once the proteins, fats, and carbs are digested, the small intestine starts to absorb them. Most of the digestion process takes place at the beginning of the small intestine and the absorption of the broken-down nutrients, water, vitamins, and minerals happens in the rest of it. Eighty percent of the water we drink is absorbed in the small intestine.

Step 6: After all the nutrients are absorbed by the small intestine, they pass into the bloodstream and are taken to your liver. Your liver processes all the nutrients, vitamins, drugs, and other things we ingest. It then turns proteins, sugar, and fat into energy, and receives help from the pancreas, which sends hormones, such as insulin, to feed the cells of your body. The liver gets rid of all the by-products from drugs and food, cholesterol, and heavy metals we don't need.

Step 7: On to the large intestine (colon), which has nothing to do with digestion, and its main job is to finish the water and electrolyte (minerals naturally found in our bodies like potassium, calcium, sodium, and magnesium) absorption that the small intestine started. The components of food that cannot be absorbed or aren't needed are excreted by the colon in the form of your poop. (GI kids)

Step 8: You POOP.

It is both complicated and amazing. The body has an exact formula that it needs to follow for your GI tract to function effectively. It connects with your hormones and nerves to communicate with and help your organs work. The GI tract contains almost as many nerves as your spinal cord, giving it its own nervous system, which gives us the chance to not worry too much when we eat. But there is room to worry when the system isn't working effectively. Because your GI tract directly feeds into your cells, organs, and body, if you are nourishing it with crap, it will treat you like crap. Your body will be in repair mode and working overtime to get rid of processed foods. For most people this can feel like bloating, exhaustion, constipation, and inflammation, plus it can affect your overall mood and energy.

I think it is so important to know what is happening in our body to become more conscious of what we put in it. If you eat something with 42 ingredients, some of which are made in labs you are making that natural process harder. The simpler we eat, the simpler this process becomes and our body thrives. If you have stomach issues, you should be aware that it can often be caused by what you are feeding it. As individualistic as we all are, the fact that we have DNA that pre-disposes us to certain foods so only you can know what works for you.

This is happening with everything you eat. Everything you put in your body.

The greater the amount of ingredients you eat means the harder your body and digestion have to work. Your body uses fluids in your stomach and organs to either acidify or alkalize the foods to extract the nutrients it needs for health. Your body gets confused when you have too much. Think about acid reflux... it is your body producing too much acid because it doesn't know what to do with what you fed it, so it sends more acid to douse it and make it usable. If you have bouts of acid reflux—your body is creating more acid to try to break food down, and your esophagus cannot keep it down. If your stomach hurts after you eat, your body is experiencing an autoimmune response, trying to repair the damage that the food you gave it caused. You need to do detective work on yourself to find what does and doesn't work for you, and in what amounts. The nutrition you eat is delivered to every one of your cells.

One thing I do to help me better understand my body is to get a colonic once a month. A colonic is literally having a professional irrigate, or pump water, into the colon to help clean it and clear it. It keeps me in check, and, as the waste from my body goes through a clear tube, I can literally see the changes in what's coming out depending on what I have been eating. Many experts in medicine and health believe that a lot of diseases start in your colon. That's why I keep going back.

Let's talk about what the body needs. Science is ever-changing as we learn more, but what we know now is that the human body has nutritional needs. When the system isn't working, you experience inflammation.

On Inflammation

On the outside of our bodies, inflammation is a physical condition in which part of the body becomes red, swollen, hot, and often painful, especially as a reaction to injury or infection in a localized area.

On the inside of our bodies, inflammation is a process in which your body's white blood cells and the things they produce protect you from infection by outside invaders, such as bacteria and viruses. But what if they are also trying to protect you from something else?

Inflammation can also be caused by your body's reaction to food. You can't have chronic inflammation and be in health. It's your body trying to repair what isn't right.

Many animal-based foods are known to cause inflammation. In 2019, the documentary "The Game Changers" premiered on Netflix (as of 2023 it is still available). What was so important was that they were able to show how your body goes into an anti-inflammatory response when you ingest animal products as opposed to plant-based ones. (Ron)

The Mind Body Medicine Center studied the benefits of plant-based foods and discovered that:

"Eating plants also combats the inflammation caused by animal foods (26,34). Therefore, decreasing animal foods while increasing plant foods has a dual effect: it not only replaces pro-inflammatory compounds with anti-inflammatory ones, but also frees up the beneficial plant compounds to address the inflammation caused by exercise, injury, and sickness."

I am a testament to the healing power of plants. Not only did my body heal from endometriosis, my recurring kidney stones disappeared as well. In February 2021 I slipped, fell, and broke my wrist in four places. It was bad. The pain was intense, and I was faced with the fact that I would need surgery to put my dominant wrist back together with metal and screws. I was worried that I would never be able to do yoga, or possibly use a chef's knife again. I was using my left hand for everything, including the writing of the beginning of this book. After this experience, I know for sure that our bodies want to heal. We need to give them the best tools possible to do it. What we eat directly feeds and nourishes our cells, and in turn supports our immune systems, our autoimmune responses, and the inflammation in our bodies.

I'm not going to say that the healing process after surgery wasn't hard, but the more time that passed, I saw that healing was possible. I couldn't do it on my own, I obviously needed my surgeon and physical therapist. My physical therapist said that all of her vegetarian and vegan clients heal so much better than the clients that ate meat, because of the inflammation factor. By May 2021, I was back to practicing planks and headstands. I know other people who have had similar injuries, but are still struggling with the healing process and inflammation years later. There are signs that our bodies need more plants to help heal, it's our job to see the connection, and take the next step.

Working with Microorganisms

It's like a busy city, looking under a microscope at your microbiome. Inside our bodies there are trillions of microbes (microorganisms). Most are in your small and large intestine but they can be found everywhere in the body. The intestine is labeled a supporting organ because it is so important. All different species, bacteria, fungus, parasites, and viruses coexist peacefully when you are healthy.

An interesting thing is that science thinks that it is passed down through your mother and her milk. So, everyone's microbiome is a little different in terms of your needs according to your DNA. This can change with lifestyle and diet over time. Normally you have more beneficial microbes than pathogens (disease), but when this number is out of balance, your health suffers.

Microorganisms help break down toxins in food and medicine, synthesize certain vitamins so your body can use them (Vitamin B12 and K), and can protect you from contaminated drinking water. It helps break down fiber and waste in the large intestine that other parts of your body couldn't. Let's just say that these little microorganisms are very important. When I started eating healthy, my microbiome went back to working for me and not against me. Eat foods that have good bacteria (like sauerkraut, pickles, and plant-based yogurts) on top of a healthy diet. Eat fermented or probiotic foods to help it get back in balance. (The micro biome)

On Hunger

Do you find yourself eating until you're full, only to feel hungry a few hours later? Do you find you're hungrier than other people? That's a sign that your body isn't looking for sustenance, it is looking for nutrients. It is literally your body's system alerting you that you are missing something in your diet. People who eat the same foods over and over again will feel this way and it can lead to disease and obesity because the body isn't getting the nutrients it needs, and its nutrient store is depleted.

For me personally, I started to realize, as I ate more and more organic plant foods, that I was less and less hungry. I didn't need to run to the fridge for late night snacks. Your body is begging you for the nutrients, it needs for energy. Do the foods you choose look like things that will give you energy? Do your foods look like they are full of vitality and life? If you are living off of indulgence your body is struggling to function, and it is letting you know. The stomach is the "second brain." Look at your gut health. It will send you signals.

One of the reasons that so many people are constantly hungry is because of their gut health. If you eat an overabundance of poor-quality foods, your gastrointestinal tract puts up defenses to protect it from the shit ingredients, like high-fructose corn syrup, sodium nitrates, and partially or fully hydrogenated oils. One of these physical defenses is called mucoid plaque. Mucoid plaque is your body's immune response to give itself an extra layer of lining when you are feeding it ingredients that it does not recognize and struggles to process.

Unfortunately, this also means that the good nutrients can't get through to our cells, and we never feel satiated as our body is looking for those ingredients. Depending on where you are in this process of divorcing your diet, it may take a few weeks for your body to trust you enough to put down these defenses and lower the wall, allowing it to take in nutrition. At the beginning of this process, the goal is to incorporate as many quality, organic, plant-based foods as possible. Literally boosting your body with as many nutrients as possible. My favorite way to do this is by drinking a daily smoothie (see the recipes in this book).

The Nutrition

In 2023, most of the 23 million search results on "what humans need nutritionally" agree. Even though the science behind food and dieting is ever-changing, these 6, or possibly 7, essential nutrients (water, carbohydrates, protein amino acids, fats, vitamins, minerals, and now some say omega-3s) have remained unchanged. In order to live a life full of vitality and energy, and to have the healthy body you want, you should first know what nutrients give your body the energy you need to take on the day.

I never really thought about food being energy before I started learning about food and feeling healthy. I guess Popeye knew all along, when he needed power, he ate spinach. I did not know this, I ate for taste, pleasure, hunger, or to control my weight growing up. I didn't eat for energy. I remember feeling dragged

down most of the time. I would want to nap after I ate. Normally, I try to eat foods that, if nothing else, don't deplete my energy.
When I started eating healthier, I noticed spikes in my energy. I
started to see that certain foods made me tired, while other foods
gave me enough energy to take on my busy life.

I remember one of my friends brought me back two vegan donuts from a big donut chain on Maui. We don't have the chain on
the island I live on, so it was a huge treat. My friend had gone out
of her way to bring me these sweet treats. As I pulled up at work,
with so much to do, I devoured both of the donuts. They were so
good to my taste buds. I licked my fingers and savored every bite.
I soon realized that even though they tasted amazing, they were so
horrible for my energy. Before I ate them, I felt fine, I was ready to
work hard. Ten minutes after eating them I had to go to my car to
take a nap, and I am not a napper. Those two donuts literally
drained me of all my energy. The quality of the ingredients in these
donuts (refined white sugars, white flours, and hydrogenated oils)
made me feel horrible. I have not enjoyed this donut chain since
then. I went from feeling good to bad in 10 minutes. The connection to this feeling was the donuts. I have enjoyed vegan donuts
since then, just not from this chain. You can buy or make quality
vegan donuts with great ingredients, like maple syrup, homemade
jams, organic flour, etc. Ingredients make the difference.

The busier I got, the more I started to eat for what I needed to
accomplish. If I am crazy busy and I have a schedule that needs
all of me, I only eat for energy. If any food may bog me down, I
avoid it. This isn't always the case, but it amazes me every time I
eat strictly for energy. FOOD IS ENERGY. Most of the time I try
to eat balanced and enjoy treats, but I choose ones that add to my
energy and don't take it away. It is amazing to discover that when
you are tired, certain foods can wake you up and give you energy.
And I don't mean coffee or energy drinks.

In order to achieve your goals, whether it be weight loss, a change in mindset, or helping to alleviate pain and inflammation, you need energy. Energy was the greatest surprise by-product of me divorcing my diet. Many humans eat to either feel good or lose weight, but after years of practice, learning how to control my energy through food was my key to solving these problems.

Before we break down nutrition, let's break down the word nutrient.

nu·tri·ent
noun
A substance that provides nourishment essential for growth and the maintenance of life.

These are the essential nutrients that our bodies need...

1. Water

Water is life. It is needed by the body for hydration, waste removal, and to regulate your temperature. It is absolutely essential for every cell in your body. You want to drink enough water for you and find that balance of how much water you need to be hydrated. See ways to stay hydrated in chapter 4 "How I Eat and Think."

2. Carbohydrates

Aka carbs. Carbohydrates are broken down into glucose, the main fuel for your body and brain. Whole food carb options include quinoa, oats, potatoes, beets, and all fruits. Complex carbs take longer to break down (e.g., sweet potato) and keep you fuller. Simple carbs (white sugar and white flour foods) break down faster and send a rush of glucose to your cells. Carbohydrates ensure you don't break down proteins to gain energy and lose muscle mass. When I eat in balance, carbs give me life. You've been told you don't need them from diet slingers, but more and more the scientific evidence is saying you need them for sustainable health.

3. Protein-Amino Acids

Protein, protein, protein. It's all you hear about these days, especially if you are vegan. Within seconds of learning that I am vegan, most people ask me where I get my protein from. The problem is that 4 out of every 5 people who ask me about it, don't know what protein is.

Proteins are made up of amino acids, which are small building blocks to life. They build our cells. They help us regulate many functions in the body. The body needs 20 different amino acids to grow and work properly. Nine of the amino acids that your body can't produce need to come from food. So, when we are talking about protein we are talking about the 9 essential amino acids we need from food. Each of these amino acids have their own functions. Some help with muscle development. Some with hair growth. Some with digestion. Some help regulate your mood.

Here are the 9 essential amino acids you need, and you may have even heard of a few of them:

Histidine, isoleucine, leucine, lysine, methionine, phenylalanine, threonine, tryptophan, valine

The current state of belief on eating animals is that it is the only way to get all of these. This isn't necessarily true. We also believe that plants can't give us complete proteins. However, I and hundreds of thousands of others, are living proof that you can. You can not only survive, but thrive.

Even though there are some amino acids that haven't been fully researched, eating a varied diet with a high amount of plants will ensure that you get the benefits from those different amino acids. When you look at nature, there aren't that many mistakes. Those amino acids are there for a reason.

Fortunately, science is catching up. Even though most plants do not have all nine amino acids, soy, buckwheat, and quinoa do. We used to think that you had to combine the other incomplete proteins to create a complete protein. Like combining rice with beans in the same meal. We have learned that your body can take, store, and use these proteins to get your daily needs met. Meaning you do not have to eat them at the same time. Getting your protein from plant sources can result in a drastic change on your health as plant proteins also give you fiber, antioxidants, minerals, vitamins, and other nutrients that we need more of in our diet. (Lee)

4. Fat

Fat is another essential nutrient that helps the absorption of vitamins and helps protect other organs.

Not all fats are created equal. Some types of fats are bad. Trans fats, found in processed foods and baked foods, as well as meat and dairy, are associated with a higher risk of heart disease and should be eaten in moderation. In natural sources, such as nuts, avocado, and some oils, unsaturated fats can protect the heart and prevent heart disease.

5. Vitamins

Vitamins are organic compounds and micronutrients that the body needs in small amounts. There isn't one food that supplies all of the vitamins we need and the amounts we need vary. Some are stored in fat to use later and others are water soluble. We need a steady stream of them coming into our bodies. Whole food sources are the best way to get vitamins and you can supplement daily with vitamin pills if you think your needs aren't being met. It's important to remember that too much of a good thing isn't a good thing. If you do decide to supplement, make sure they are organic, and the cleanest supplements you can buy.

Here is a list of the essential vitamins and what they help your body with:

- Vitamin A. Skin and eye health. Helps keep skin and membranes healthy. Boosts the immune system and its functions. Plant sources include: yams, sweet potatoes, broccoli, spinach, red bell pepper, apricots.
- Vitamin C. Bone, muscle structure, and immune support. Essential for preventing infections by creating antibodies. Plant sources include: kiwi, kale, all citrus, red bell pepper, strawberries, papayas.
- Vitamin D. Bone growth, cardiovascular, nervous system health, bone growth, and immune health. Helps to boost energy from within the cell. A hormone normally produced in the skin using energy from sunlight, vitamin D can also be found in a few foods—but is best from sunlight—and can also be effectively boosted with vitamin D supplements.
- Vitamin E. Works as an antioxidant to build healthy cells. It neutralizes free radicals. Plant sources include: sunflower oil, safflower oil, sunflower seeds, hazelnuts, almonds, and peanut butter.
- Vitamins B-6 and 12. Convert foods into energy (metabolism), create new blood cells, and maintains healthy skin cells, brain cells, and other body tissues. All B vitamins are essential, but

6 and 12 have important functions when it comes to immune health. Plant sources include: carrots, spinach, and sweet potatoes. These all contain vitamin B-6. B-12 is more commonly found in meat and dairy, but healthier options with B-12 are fortified non-dairy milk and nutritional yeast.

I am not a scientist, not a doctor, or a nutritionist. I am a mom of three, a vegan chef, and a health coach. After watching my mom die in a hospital at the mercy of doctors, I made a pledge to learn to tend to my temple. To know my body better than my doctor. I also don't pretend to know what a doctor knows, their knowledge is so vast. However, I put the responsibility on myself to learn what makes my body optimal, so I'm less dependent on doctors. Doctors study disease, I study health. I also believe we have the ability to turn disease on and off. I have read books on all types of diets, lifestyles, and nutrition over the last 13 years. Our bodies love to heal and be in health, they just need help from us. Our choices are a supporting role with our body being the star.

One important part of health is supplementing your body with vitamins, minerals, and nutrition. Every vitamin supports a system or another vitamin that supports a system. After all of my research, these are my go-to, immune-boosting, virus, and bacteria-fighting gems. I go heavy on vitamins, and then take a break, so my body can use what it has stored.

6. Minerals

Minerals are another essential nutrient. Each mineral has its own function in your body.

Seven essential minerals are: sodium, iron, potassium, calcium, magnesium, zinc, and phosphorus. Minerals are essential for bone health, muscle and nerve function, and circulation. They are also needed to keep nerves and muscles working correctly.

- Folate. Most known for being essential during pregnancy. Folate is still a must-have. It's involved in multiple life-sustaining processes, including DNA synthesis. Without enough folate, the neurotransmitters that regulate your mood get lazy. Not enough folate means not enough red blood cells, which may affect your energy levels. Plant sources include: dark, leafy green veggies like kale and spinach, as well as asparagus and brussels sprouts.
- Selenium. Selenium may be the most underestimated nutrient when it comes to defending against viruses. It helps to produce more T-cells. Plant sources include: Brazil nuts, sunflower seeds, grains.
- Zinc. Zinc is responsible for antibody production. It promotes wound healing. Plant sources include: whole grains, nuts, seeds, beans. (White)

And last but not least, the newest addition to the list:

7. Omega-3 fatty acids

Omega-3 fatty acids increase brain health and may help heart function. Your body can't create omega-3, so you must have sources of it in your diet. They are essential for heart health, cell functions, and hormone production. Omega-3 can reduce inflammation and minimize the risk of heart disease and stroke. Plant sources include: nuts (like walnuts and hazelnuts) and seeds (flaxseeds). (Amos)

Our bodies have needs. The question is—are you giving it what it needs to function optimally? We as individuals have differing needs, daily, weekly, and monthly. We need a varied diet, and plants and fruits offer more variety of all these things.

Animals and animal foods offer a lot of nutrition because the animals have needs close to ours to sustain life. They don't even have everything, and with factory farming they are fed soy and corn and grass that has been sprayed with pesticides. They are given antibiotics too. When you eat them you need to get rid of all their toxins through your body. You can get more from a varied plant diet, whether you eat animals or not. Each fruit and vegetable is its own vitamin, full of nutrition, in the right amount for your body's needs. Are you getting a multi vitamin of food?

Also, look at:

- Probiotics/prebiotics. Studies are showing that health starts in the gut and that there are millions of bacteria that help us break down and process nutrition from food. (Fields) Anytime my tummy is off, I dose myself with pre/probiotics. As opposed to taking another pill, I rely on fermented products. I depend on Synergy products like kombucha, water kefir, and fermented plant-based yogurts. These are raw and living foods. I count on products that cultivate living probiotics. I love the products so much that I became friends with the founder, GT Dave and I have seen firsthand that he practices what he preaches. A common-sense caution—choose companies that are in it for your health, like Synergy™.

As I stated before, I'm no professional, but I do believe that all of these nutrients can help nourish your cells, and boost your immune system defenses. Many vitamins, hormones, and minerals are needed for health. Each and every one helps a different vitamin, hormone, or mineral to function. So if you are low on one, it can contribute to different functions of the body not working. So stock up, start a routine, keep a journal on what you're taking, and see if you feel different. We have the power to not only prevent disease by having a healthy system, but we also have the ability to help our bodies heal when in disease. And if you are concerned, get a blood test that shows you what you need. Work with a naturopath or doctor to figure it out.

Now that we have a better understanding that the mind, body, and nutrition are interconnected, let's deep dive into some of the food beliefs that are holding you back.

You are a constantly
changing and evolving
human.

Chapter 3

BREAK UP WITH YOUR
FOOD BELIEFS

Biggest Belief I Broke Up With—Health Is Not a Given

What worked for you in the past won't always work for you now, because you are different. You are a constantly changing and evolving human.

As you learned in the last chapter, our bodies are tricky to say the least. Our relationship with food is a completely symbiotic one. Your body has needs, and certain foods help fulfill those needs. Your body needs a certain amount of vitamins, minerals, fats, carbs, proteins, and water. Those needs are changing constantly based on what we have stored and what we are eating. Oftentimes, we will start a diet or cleanse and feel really good and see changes, and then we plateau. We also need to be aware that when we start a diet or cleanse, we have a different set of needs than the previous one we attempted. To make it more complicated, your needs change based on your age, stress levels, and overall health. All of the nutrients you need also work together to support processes in the body and our basic life functions. So, if you're low on one thing, like iron or vitamin C, your body may not be able to function as well or run these processes as smoothly, even if it has everything else it needs. The systems in your body are totally symbiotic, and they work together to do the best they can for you. In return, they need the best fuel you can provide.

There are so many diets out there, but there is only one YOU. If we changed the amount of time we spend trying to figure out someone else's diet and took that time to learn about you, you would find health. You need to focus on your needs. Many times the authors of books don't follow what they propose, but you feel defeated if you can't keep up. These diets we are trying to split up with are selling us a false promise. Those false promises aren't good for our bodies or our brains. We also store knowledge of all these diets as facts and they become our food beliefs, like how some people believe carbohydrates make them gain weight, or that all sugar is bad, or that we need to drink animal milk for calcium. We start this at a very young age, and it can be hard to separate the truth from the fiction.

One of the goals of reading this book is finding what foods do and don't support you in becoming your best self. The you that is living in health, with vitality and energy. You can't do it holding onto beliefs from the past. Hopefully, the last chapter taught you there is so much to our relationships with food and our bodies.

One of the biggest things you can do for yourself to find health is to re-learn some beliefs you have about food.

When I first went vegan, I started noticing that many past beliefs I had about food weren't true. They were actually the opposite. I had held on to those beliefs for a long time. I'll give you an example. I thought a calorie was a calorie, and eating healthier meant eating fewer calories. What I found is the opposite: a large orange and 1 store-bought cookie have almost the same amount of calories. But one is much different. By just looking at their calories we equate them in terms of their benefits to our body. But if you break them down, and look at the nutrients they have, they aren't equals. Even a child could look at an orange and a cookie and tell you which is healthier.

I also saw the amount of healthy food I could eat for calories. The portions went up in size, calorie for calorie. A lot of the advice you get just tells you to eat less of the same foods, but never addresses the quality of the ingredients and the impact that chemicals have on our health. I was surprised when I noticed I was able to eat more plant-based foods, and feel fuller, calorie for calorie.

As I started cleansing and listening to others' advice, I would take it on as fact.

When the natural sugars in fruit became the enemy a few years ago (many high protein–low sugar diets suggest little to no fruit), I followed the fad. I stopped having fruit and when I did, I thought all fruit was bad for me. What I learned is that sometimes my body likes short term breaks from fruit, but in the long term, fruit is good for my body.

It took me years to let go of some of my beliefs and I am still working through the stubborn ones. It is also important to remember that I am constantly forming new beliefs that may not serve me in the future, and that I will have to break up with beliefs for the rest of my life because life is ever changing.

Now, it's your turn. Let's break up with your beliefs that no longer serve you or your body. Let's be open to seeing how our body feels. What are your beliefs around food?

1. Do you eat for energy or pleasure?

2. What were/are your habits around food?

3. What habits did you learn growing up around food?

4. What are three truths you have about food?

5. How many times do you eat when you're not hungry?

After you answer these questions, determine whether your answers have a positive, negative, or neutral impact on your health. This also gives you the opportunity to think about where your beliefs about food came from.

Even though I can't see your answers, I do know from working with hundreds of people that we all have 1 or 2 negative answers, and that they may vary by person.

Growing up in my house, food wasn't eaten for its nutrition, but rather to keep the kids full. We didn't drink water, even when we worked out. I also ate sugary cereal as a meal more than a few times. All of this seemed normal to me. Even though I became a vegetarian at a young age, I still believed you needed dairy to do your body good. These were some of my limiting beliefs. I had to break up with these and face the fact that I was not healthy, and the foods I was eating were not helping.

I want you to see the reality of food instead of the illusion that comes from your beliefs.

If you notice that any of your answers to the questions are holding you back from adopting a new lifestyle, or cause an inability to try new things, you need to let them go and see what waits for you on the other side. Now is the time to break up with that belief.

There are a few habits I have used to divorce my diet and let go of things that didn't serve me in the past. When I need to adjust my food beliefs, this is what I do...

1. I ask if it is going to bring ease to my health or disease to my health. If the answer is disease, 9 times out of 10 I opt to not eat it. Notice I said 9. I'm not perfect, and I don't want to lead you to believe I am.

2. I ask myself what have I done for my body today. If I can't answer, I drink water or eat something healthy. I need reminders hourly and daily to take care of myself. With how stretched thin we are these days, it is very normal in society to take care of our health and our needs last.

3. Try to do the opposite of what you think. If you think fruit is too sugary or bad for you, try fruit in the morning and actually see how you feel. These beliefs are so limiting and can keep us from our full health potential.

4. Eat healthfully until you feel full. Don't think of portion size, eat healthy foods in abundance until you feel full. When in doubt, add more organic veggies.

5. Every time you have cravings for something that doesn't serve you mentally or physically, make a yummy smoothie

or protein shake. Wait 20 minutes and see if you still have the craving. More often than not you won't want the unhealthy snack.

Following these steps can help you BREAK UP with whatever beliefs aren't serving you.

I have three fundamentals
for health:

1. Eat more vegan or plant-based
2. Eat organic
3. Drink more water

If you do nothing else but adopt
these three habits in your life,
you will see DRAMATIC changes
to your health.

I myself experienced this. These three keys are the roadmap I have used to find and sustain health. They are my guiding star when I lose it and need to find it again.

It took me years to do this, but there were so many things I learned about myself, and I have learned that so many of other people's ideas were wrong for me. Here are some examples of some diets I tried, and why I had to let them and my beliefs around them go:

1. Gluten-Free: Obviously if you have celiac disease or are unable to process gluten, you should not eat gluten. However, I tried a gluten-free diet, even though I was not gluten intolerant. Was cutting gluten good for me? No! It turns out I was just eating the wrong types of gluten and not taking seasonal breaks from it. Of course white bread filled with sugar is going to be crap for your body, same with those cookies that are made with conventional processed, bleached flour. If you have a better understanding of the ingredients, you can look for more options that are made with organic flours.

2. Cut Carbs: After trying gluten-free I thought maybe the issue could have been starchy carbohydrates like white rice and potatoes. Cutting and replacing potatoes from my life didn't help. In fact, I got rid of a powerhouse vegetable that helps me stay fuller and in health. I can eat so many potatoes and not gain weight. I am meant for them or they are meant for me. Obviously it can depend on how you make your potatoes, but remember it is all about your ingredients! Organic baked potato fries will always be healthier than fast food 6 ingredient "French Fries."

3. Sugar-Free: What is true for potatoes is also true here. Sugar isn't the culprit, but the type of sugar and amount you are ingesting may be. High fructose corn syrup is used to sweeten so many packaged products. When I add a moderate amount of organic cane sugar or maple syrup to my baked goods and coffee, I still feel good.

4. Thinking that it was one thing. Too much fat, too much sugar, too much protein, or not enough. Health for me is about finding balance now. Not a yoyo that makes one thing the culprit. Unless I have an allergy to a food that is fucking up my system, if I eat a whole food diet while being mindful, I can enjoy it all.

I have had to look at what I thought I knew and be willing to disregard it. One time, while I was traveling as a vegan in Italy, I had been on a carb-free, grain-free, and fruit-free diet for a few months. Initially I had lost weight, but 10 pounds kept sticking on. I didn't feel good. While I was traveling around beautiful Italy, I had to survive on carbs like pasta, bread, and pizzas (without the cheese).

Traveling while eating vegan, I had to eat carbs, pasta, bread, pizza, and all of the fruit—and guess what?

I felt so good. I had been carbohydrate starved, however if I kept eating that way when I returned from my trip, I would have had too many carbs. It's a balance to find what makes you feel good and when. As you learned in chapter 2, your body needs all of the nutrients. How much of what you need is up to what your body's needs are presently.

Of any of the things I do for my health, food still has the biggest impact. Most of us are making daily choices based on our taste buds, and not how they are making us feel physically.

Remember, food is energy, make no mistake. What you are fueling up on is fueling you. Do you notice how you feel after certain foods? That's your body's ability to tell you at that moment if a food is working for you and if it isn't. Feeling overfull, wanting to take a nap, and getting bloated aren't processes the body relies on. That's an alarm system from your body telling you that what you ate didn't work for it. Yes, there are foods that are worth this feeling every once in a while, like overloading on French fries when out with friends, eating donuts by yourself (is this only me?), or whatever your indulgence is. If this is how you feel most of the time, it's not you, it's the FOOD.

Do you find it difficult to stay on one diet? Are you confused by the amount of different information?

Health is something that evades most of us. Some of us feel it short-term, but don't have the tools to make it last long-term. At times, I have my physical health in check, but emotionally I suffer. Other times, it's the reverse. True health is when we feel healthy physically and emotionally, body and mind—true soul alignment. I have a friend that calls it "tending the temple." To take care of our temple. To find true health in a manageable time that fits into our lifestyle. This is a piece I see missing in most of the information out there. Such rigid plans that don't meet us where we are at, and don't address our goals or lifestyle. They also only focus on one piece, either physical health OR emotional health, but without both of these, it's hard to feel healthy.

Health is an evolution. I have had to try so many diets and cleanses and what I have found is that if it doesn't fit into my busy life, it won't work long term. During that time, I owned a restaurant and wrote a cookbook, all as a mom to three. All the while, trying to make the best choices for my family and my health. I don't have a lot of extra time and what I found was that while I was trying to cleanse myself and feed my family, if there wasn't balance, I was lucky if it lasted two weeks.

I found myself at one point in my best body health. I was working out, eating so well, and my body showed it. My mind and emotions felt so low at that point. I felt so incongruent and I didn't feel healthy. I remember thinking, "At least you're a skinny bitch." I knew I was missing something, and one day, while on my closet floor crying, I decided I would invest in me. The whole ME. I dove deep into myself. I found myself. I felt healthy inside and out. Then I lost it, then I would get it back. I finally had an AHA moment when I fell out of true health, and asked, "What can I do to realign it?"

I realized true health is not only practical, it's a PRACTICE. I have to be in it. I have to create time for health as a practice. I need reminders. I need it to be sustainable, practical, and manageable. This exercise is a health practice and provides easy ways to tend to your physical and emotional health. I created it for me, as well as you, it is my daily practice.

The Check-In Tool

Let me introduce you to the check-in tool.

Check in with yourself every day. You can do this in a journal or in your notes on your phone. I do it at night before bed. You can also do it in the morning the day after. This is an amazing tool for keeping track of how you feel and what you eat. You may start to see some links between not feeling good and a certain food.

Jot down a short menu of what you ate during the day.

Then ask yourself...

1. How do you feel overall?
2. Did you feel overfull? Content? Hungry?
3. How was your mood?
4. How was your energy?
5. Any symptoms?

Here is an example:

Today I had:
- a smoothie (choc, pb, banana)
- a salad (greens, nutritional yeast, lemon)
- a pear
- a protein bar (choc)
- Bean and cheese burritos (beans, vegan cheese, salad)
- a brownie (g-free)

We want to be able to look at links and symptoms at the end of the day. This just becomes an intuitive practice after a while. When you are in health, you can handle a few hits. If there are too many hits, then your body is out of health. If a glass of wine, a beer, or cocktail does knock you out of balance, then you need to give yourself a little break and regain your balance. I talk about this more at the end of chapter 4 when I discuss the importance of resetting. Also, keeping notes on how you eat and how you feel shows you real proof of why you need to break up with beliefs and helps shine a spotlight on what your new beliefs should be. You are leading the science experiment to determine the keys to your health.

Back to the Greek father of medicine, Hippocrates, whose principles of medicine are still used today. He had quite a bit to say. You might be asking yourself what does an Ancient Greek doctor have to do with health today? All I know is that my findings on healing align with a lot of what he talked about then. More so than any doctor I have spoken to. The second I realized food was my key to health, I noticed the changes in my body, and became more intuitive about myself. The ancients were focused on health care (healing) and not sick care like we are now. How many of us have had loved ones who have gotten sick, and then sicker as they tried many different cures? This isn't to say that there aren't cures to be found and cures that work, but the first step should always be to take a look at what we are putting into our bodies on a daily basis.

Here is a meaningful quote from Hippocrates…

"If we could give every individual the right amount of nourishment and exercise, not too little and not too much, we would have found the safest way to health."

Food heals, nutrients heal, not too little and not too much of either. Our lives are all about balance. Are you ready to find that balance and give up everything you think you know about food? Are you ready to adopt some healthier habits using ingredients that are more natural than what you are eating now? If not, here's more reasons why you may want to.

Eating well is a form of self-respect

What is in your food? Additives in Food

Ingredients are the most important information on the nutritional label. Read that again. Ignore the values and read the ingredients. It tells you a lot about the quality.

I know from having my products on the shelf when I had a wholesale baking company, that the FDA requires ingredient labels to be listed from the most to the fewest ingredients.

For example, here are the ingredients of blueberry muffins from a chain grocery store in the United States.

Enriched Bleached Flour (Wheat Flour, Niacin, Ferrous Sulfate, Thiamine Mononitrate, Riboflavin, Folic Acid), Sugar, Water, Soybean Oil, Blueberries, Eggs, Modified Corn Starch, Contains 2% or Less of: Partially Hydrogenated Shortening (Soybean Oil, Cottonseed, or Canola Oil, Propylene Glycol Mono- and Diesters of Fatty Acids, Mono and Diglycerides, Soy Lecithin, BHT), Emulsifier (Propylene Glycol Monoesters, Monoglycerides, Sodium Stearoyl Lactylate), Salt, Nonfat Milk, Sodium Bicarbonate, Sodium Aluminum Phosphate, Cellulose Gum, Artificial Flavor, Sodium Caseinate, Guar Gum, Xanthan Gum.

About seven of those ingredients are recognizable. Seven out of 19. Of those ingredients there are so many additives to improve flavor, texture, and shelf life. There is more sugar than water and blueberries.

It isn't just grocery stores—here are the ingredients to blueberry muffins from a warehouse big box store.

CakeMix (Flour, Sugar, Vegetable Oil) Baking Powder, Salt, Shortening (Palm or Palm Kernel Oil, Canola and Modified Palm Oils, Dextrose, Artificial Flavor, Dry Skim Milk, Dried Albumen, Yeast, Citric Acid, Xanthan Gum, Sodium Stearoyl, Lactate, Sodium Aluminum Phosphate, Mono and Diglycerides), Blueberries, Liquid Albumen and Yolk, Canola Oil, Water, Flour

All their recipes for baked goods start with their cake mix. Also, notice that blueberries are almost at the end of the ingredient list. That means there are not a lot of blueberries. One more ingredient I want to point out to you is "dextrose." This is a sugar made from corn or wheat, usually genetically modified and sprayed with pesticides. It's fake sugar.

Why should we care? Your poor body has to break all this down and figure out what to do with those ingredients. It is trying to separate the nutrients from the ingredients and process what it needs, but this process becomes more and more difficult when you eat foods with so many conventional ingredients, half of which aren't actual food.

To give you an idea of how simple this could be, here is my blueberry muffin recipe, and keep in mind, I used to sell these at my restaurant and at local grocery stores on Kauai.

Organic Flour, Organic Sugar (White, Coconut, or Maple), Baking Soda, Baking Powder, Salt, Organic Almond Milk, Organic Blueberries, Organic Olive Oil

What is easier on your body? Eight easy to break down ingredients, or 19–25 unrecognizable ones? Remember, many grocery stores and bakeries don't have to list what pesticides come with your non-organic, not freshly baked store version.

In the past 50 years, food has become about how easy it is, how fast it is to acquire, and how best to market to you. Most foods contain enriching agents that aren't good for your body because your body has no use for them. Softeners are added to most packaged breads and baked goods, because normal bread goes stale. This additive makes your flour softer and makes it melt in your mouth as if it were freshly baked, even though it's not. That does not sound yummy.

I don't know about you but I don't want all those additives in my food. Do these giant food companies care about your health? No! They care about their sales and tricking your taste buds to want more and more of their foods. They enrich crappy foods with crappy vitamins and minerals, and lead you to believe that you are doing good things for your body. Take a look, if the nutrition from your food comes from additives it's not really good nutrition.

Most of enriched packaged foods, like flours, cereals, or snack foods, have additives because these foods have very little actual nutrition. They are trying to add the nutrients in. Real whole foods don't need to have added nutrients. If for some reason you aren't completely getting the nutrients you need, due to an allergy or something else, there are definitely better-quality nutrients than the ones that big companies are adding to their white breads. Why do we want to make nutritionally devoid foods have nutrients, all the while making the puzzle pieces harder to put back together and separate in our body's digestive system?

I personally don't want some bioengineered gross vitamins and minerals blasted into my bread or cereal to trick me into thinking it's healthy. When I eat bread, pasta, snacks, or any high-carb, yet low-nutrition product, that is what I'm getting, filler food. To me a filler food is anything that is low in nutrition compared to a whole food. I don't want my chips to have protein and vitamins added to them. There are times I have a protein shake or a protein bar, as a meal replacement. However, we have taken these ideas and now are starting to sprinkle them over unhealthy foods to trick us into believing they are healthy.

I met a woman looking for almond milk at the store. She was looking so perplexed and asked me why the brands with a lot of ingredients have calcium and the ones with just water and almonds don't. I tried to explain to her that companies add vitamins and calcium to their milk. Almonds have nutrition, but when you make them into milk, you are diluting it, so it is not crazy nutritious. I told her to get the simple milk and get a high-end calcium supplement. She told me her doctor said not to get a pill, but to get non-dairy milk with it added. She nor her doctor understood that it's added vitamins and they are not the most bio available high quality vitamins. I personally would rather supplement with the best, highest quality supplement pill, than with an additive.

I also have friends that love protein with everything, but don't even know what it is. As we add protein and nutrients to food, we are ignoring the difference between alive, vital whole foods and powder-blasted food. There is a difference. A big difference. Don't let marketing fool you, shit foods with protein and vitamins blasted on them are still shit foods.

General Rule, "If you don't know what it is, don't buy it."

Animals

I have a question for you, how many animals do you eat?

The numbers are staggering but the average person (non-vegetarian) in the United States eats 174 animals a year. I think most people mentally minimize how much meat, eggs, and dairy they eat. Oftentimes, when I am working with new clients or having lunch with friends, they tell me they barely eat animals, but I notice that they eat animals with every meal. It's in the butter on your veggies, the eggs on your toast, the cheese sprinkled in your salad. I don't want to shame you, or to point a finger, but with awareness we start to see things for how they really are. I'm just inviting you to look at it. For the most part, I don't even like speaking to people about it, because it's such a hot button topic. A lot of times, meat lovers need to tell me, after they find out I'm vegan, why they need to eat meat. I hate arguing with people and try to back out of the conversation.

I don't know what is right for you, or anyone, or what's right for the world. Eating more plant-based foods and less meat is better for most people, better for animals, and proven research has shown that it's better for planet Earth. It's really a no brainer, look at nature and see how much abundance there is in the plant world, even without human intervention.

Look at nature. Plants grow and are much more abundant than animals. I live in Hawaii and abundantly see everything. When the avocado tree is in season, it is dripping in avocados. They are easy to get and collect. Same with mango. Cherry tomatoes grow wild by the thousands. Citrus is crazy abundant. Animals not so much. I see wild pigs and chickens here and there. However, if you aren't actively hunting them, you won't see them very often. I walk all the time. The island I live on has chickens running free everywhere, but I have never seen an egg in the wild. Not once. It has forced me to see that if you look at nature, you will see that all the answers are there.

Today, I opened a papaya, and to my delight, it was full of seeds, like almost all fruits and veggies. If I didn't go to the store and actually grew my own food, each organic vegetable and fruit can become many more vegetables or fruit. If you dry the seeds you can plant them the next season and ensure you have plenty of fruit and vegetables. Many animals on the other hand have gestations closer to humans. They have to be raised to be able to become your food. To me, if you look at life a little more naturally, you will see we were meant to mainly eat plants and fruits. More than you probably think. Think about it, every fruit and vegetable you eat comes with a way to propagate it.

You may eat way more animals than you are aware of, and it's time to look at this. Especially if there is a chance that animal products are causing inflammation and disease in your body. We are a society that is not in moderation or balance when it comes to animal products. I am not here to tell you that you can't eat meat, but that adding more plants and eating less meat will improve your health overall. Don't believe me? Try it for yourself.

According to a study completed in 2015 by the Vegetarian Calculator group (vegeratiancalculator.com) the average meat eater will eat around 7000 animals in their lifetime. This was widely reported at the time of the study. There are so many studies showing that animal-based foods (meat, eggs, and dairy) can cause inflammation in your body. If you are dealing with inflammation you want to become aware of how many animals you eat. I'm not saying you have to give up animal products entirely, but for you to become more aware of how much you are ingesting.

My goal with this book is to teach you to become aware of the quality of the food you intake. Personally, I don't believe that there is a need for humans to eat animals anymore. We have so many amazing, healthful options. I'm proof you can live vibrantly and happily without eating animals. But let's take it one step at a time. I'm not here to tell you to stop eating meat, but I do want you to become aware of the implications to your health from a meat heavy diet. When I first went vegan I was shocked to find how many packaged foods included animal products. Almost every meal and snack included some animal products in it. My foods weren't vibrant, organic, or healthy and as a result neither was I. The foods I was eating had a direct impact on my weight, my health, and my clarity of mind.

Maybe it's the creamer in your coffee every morning, or the cheese you put on your salad or pasta, or the bone broth you drink. The average American has dairy in their coffee, eggs served with cheese and meat, and butter on their toast. Many people add chicken to their salads or have a turkey sandwich for lunch, which usually has eggs (mayonnaise) and dairy (cheese). Maybe for dinner a burger, with more dairy and eggs (mayo), and bacon. Or perhaps a steak with potatoes that have added dairy. Maybe sushi for dinner, or salmon over rice. A diet even in the perceived "healthiest form," has animals and animal products all over it.

I urge you to track your meals for a day, and see where all of the hidden animal ingredients are. You don't have to change everything all at once, but maybe you can use olive oil instead of butter in your potatoes or on your toast. Perhaps switching over to a delicious vegan cheese or mayonnaise. I promise you won't taste the difference because vegan mayonnaise is AMAZING!

Removing these hidden animal products when you can is a benefit, not only to animals and the planet, but also your body. Once you start to take a better look at the foods you are consuming, you are one step closer to being able to see what foods have a positive and negative impact on your body. This type of intuition helps you develop a better sense of your health and also guides you when you do eat foods with less optimal ingredients.

Does milk really do a body good?

We are the only species that drinks and eats another species' milk, and the only species that continues drinking milk after childhood.

Although this amazing elixir is great when we are babies (only human milk though, remember we can't give our babies cow's milk until they are one), studies are now showing that milk and dairy consumption into adulthood can cause so many issues and diseases.

Our society has a hard time watching people nursing their babies into childhood, but they have no issue with forcing cows to nurse while we drink their milk. Not only that, but these animals are given hormones and antibiotics to help them continue producing milk, because otherwise they would naturally lose their supply. They need antibiotics because their utters are so sore and sick from overuse, and the food they are given is also genetically modified crap, which we then streamline into the form of a glass of milk. I understand the desire to search for an alternative like grass-fed cow's milk, but they are still given antibiotics. This resembles an animal hospital more than the happy farm you are picturing to justify it.

Anyway, enough with the politics of it all, I could write a whole different book on that. What I want you to think about more is the food itself, learn more about it, and how it impacts your body.

After reading Colin T. Campbell's *The China Study* when it came out in 2006, we were finally able to see scientific evidence of what is obvious, but which many choose to ignore. Eating more complex carbohydrates from fruits and vegetables are keys to weight loss, but they are also keys to our health. Protein, specifically from animals (meat and dairy), can lead to disease.

"The people who eat the most animal protein have the most heart disease, cancer, and diabetes."

(Campbell)

When we are trying to feel our best and have the most vitality there is clearly a better choice.

You need to learn to trust yourself. What do I mean by this? Science is a practice and ever changing. Yes, it's true. Science and nutrition are ever changing with the breakthroughs we learn. A lot of what you were taught at school are the food beliefs you have, or maybe it's what your parents and family taught you. Do you have a disease that just runs in the family, like diabetes or high blood pressure? Maybe it's the diet habits you have learned from your family. Let's start with the food pyramid. Did you know the food pyramid is different in other countries? Did you know it has changed over the years? Do you believe you are what you eat? Did you know we grow enough vegetables to feed 45 billion animals a year to turn into food, when we could just feed all the 9 billion beings on the planet?

I know that, for me, food has made the biggest difference in my overall health, I still have to work on it every day. It is a relationship. This takes us back to the yo-yoing of diets. Why do they work the first time but maybe not the next time?

The better question is why do we keep going back to them, like a bad relationship, thinking it will be different? It's because you are different, and yet you are hoping for the same outcomes. There is not one diet or way you could eat that would sustain you for a healthy life forever. You have to be in a relationship with food, and intuitively trust that if you are in health, you will know what you need, or try something to get you back there.

Anyway, like I said there are studies for both sides, that's why you want to divorce your diet and start learning. When I went vegan, and ate more whole plant-based foods, everything in my body changed. Only your body knows. If animal products are causing your health to decline, or cause an inflammatory response in your body, start to pay attention and see how you feel—become your own study. Did I feel better after a veggie burger than I do with a regular burger? You have to be looking to notice. Outside of animal products and the health effects of overconsumption, there are a few simple ways the world has influenced me to be more natural.

On Eating Seasonally

Our bodies exist on planet Earth. On our beautiful planet, we have seasons. Of course the weather varies depending on where you live, but for the most part, within these seasons, plants grow. It has only been in the past 100 years that we have had more access to a greater variety of food than ever before. While this can be a good thing, there can also be too much of a good thing.

I like to eat seasonally, meaning eating fruits, vegetables, and grains that are as fresh as possible, grown in a way that they thrive. This helps my body thrive. Some people say an apple a day keeps the doctor away, and while I do appreciate the sentiment, it's definitely not true. Your body can get used to food, eating the same thing like an apple when it is out of season, isn't fucking natural. Remember not too much, not too little.

The natural world is fascinating. We are literally given food to grow that comes in abundance at different times of the year. There would also be a season for cleansing, because of food shortages due to the season, though much of it stores for a longer period of time (potatoes, squash, grains, wheat), but it is also a time when we would have naturally have eaten less. The amazing thing is that all the produce in the world is like a variety of multivitamins that you need and need to store. If you eat a rainbow (meaning many different fruits and vegetables of different colors) you are getting vitamins and minerals, fats, protein, and carbs, all in a biodegradable package. I'm a big believer that because nature is in seasons and every plant and tree has a season, we should not eat everything year-round. Our bodies weren't meant for a pill a day. We are so complex and the food we have been given on this planet is also complex. So eat seasonal, even if you're out of season. SO, you could hit apple's hard in the summer, instead of fall (their season) or pumpkin in the spring, instead of winter, but make sure you give your body a rest to assimilate what it needs and stores.

Circadian Cycles

The precursor to intermittent fasting.

Circadian cycles are the cycles of our planet, from the sun rising every day, to the sun setting every evening. There are hours of both light and darkness. I believe intermittent fasting is just following our daily clock. No matter how sophisticated we become, we have a clock that is tied to this planet. Most of us sort of follow these patterns on a daily basis, we rise with the sun (again some of us) and go to sleep a few hours after the sun goes down. Around 200 years ago, we didn't really have the ability to see and cook at night, we followed the cycles. So if you want to be good to your body or give it a break, don't fast, just eat sun up until sun down. Your natural clock will thank you. This also gives our body ample time to cleanse itself instead of digesting food. This is the goal.

Organics

Did you know your coffee, if it isn't organic, doesn't just come with a jolt of caffeine, it also comes with a bunch of pesticides?

It's not just coffee, but also most fruits, veggies, grains, meats, and packaged foods that don't have to list the chemicals and fertilizers they are being grown with.

Encyclopedia Britannica states that organic food is "fresh or processed food produced by organic farming methods. Organic food is grown without the use of synthetic chemicals, such as human-made pesticides and fertilizers, and does not contain genetically modified organisms (GMOs). Organic foods include fresh produce, meats, and dairy products as well as processed foods such as crackers, drinks, and frozen meals." (ORGANIC FOOD)

Here is a list of chemicals and fertilizers in your morning cup of coffee.

Endosulfan (brand name Thiodan), chlorpyrifos (brand name Dursban), diazinon (brand name Basudin), methyl parathion (aka ethyl parathion, parathion), triadimefon (brand name Bayleton).

I could give you the reasons why they use them, but I'd rather give you the list of side effects from these which can not only cause short term symptoms like fatigue, weakness, and brain fog, but can also lead to long-term health consequences like disease, neurodegenerative disorder, and some autoimmune diseases. So many foods are highly sprayed and you don't know.

I want to talk about one pesticide in particular that is found on and in so many different foods.

Glyphosate—it's the main ingredient in weed killer and can be found in our water, air, and blood thanks to the overuse of it. Most places and food have limits on how much glyphosate is safe for us. Considering I can't control the amount in the air and water, even though I have never sprayed it in my life, I choose to not have it in my food.

Many people link gluten intolerance with the amount of gly-phosate that is sprayed on wheat. I could give you a science study, or you could try to eat only organic bread and see if you feel better. I recommend that if you want to know more, do your research.

Almost all foods grown and sold today have pesticides. We have a steady drip of it, in our coffee, breakfast foods, fruits, all snacks, vegetables, and pretty much all of your food. You can Google search and find all the pesticides that are in your products without too much effort.

Did you know there are pesticides in our bloodstream or that pesticide residue can be found in our clean, "drinkable" water? Worse still, it's been found in the umbilical cords of newborns. Eating organic and more plant-based is a partnership. It benefits our health and our environment. GMOs are in so many products in our shelves.

On GMOs

GMOs are genetically modified organisms. There is so much mis-information about GMOs. Many people think it is the mixing of the genetics of two plants like combining a nectarine and a peach. Many believe that science is creating new plants that stand up to threats from Mother Earth. However, GMOs are a little differ-ent. What these large corporations do is take the DNA of an in-secticide and splice it into the vegetable's DNA, so it grows with its own insecticide inside, and thus takes care of the bugs that eat it. The problem with that is that the concentrations of insecticide can be up to a thousand times stronger in a GMO vegetable than what you would find in the dirt.

GMO companies are chemical companies, Google it. They don't have your health at the forefront. Their goal is to make money. They have no concerns for your health or your wellness. There is a reason to be wary of putting their food into your body. Fortunately, I'm not the only one that thinks so. Many of these "conventional" GMO foods are banned in the European Union and many other countries around the world either don't allow GMOs in their food or they legally have to be labeled. Even though they are presented as "safe", in reality, we are the science experiment for GMOs, learning if a body can tolerate this amount of pesticides or different plant DNA. All I know is I don't want me or my kids to be anyone's experiment. Diseases are skyrocketing. GMOs were allowed into the food supply in 1995. I would rather err on the side of nature, and take care of myself. All organic food is non-GMO, so to me it's a no brainer. They recently had a brand re-do and the formerly known GMOs and Frankenfoods are now often referred to as bio engineered. If you have the choice, why not choose the option you know is going to be free of pesticides and GMOs?

When shopping for produce, follow the guides from produce codes. Here's my cheat sheet.

- Organic produce has a five-digit code beginning with "9."
- Conventionally grown produce four-digit code beginning with "4."
- GMO produce begins with "8."

I stay away from buying GMO foods. Sometimes it's hard to know what has it and what doesn't. The USDA has approved corn, soybeans, potatoes, squash, papayas, apples, alfalfa, and sugar beets to be genetically modified, and these are currently being grown and sold on the market. This means that almost 99% of the corn syrup or soy products you buy and consume as ingredients in your favorite products are GMO. Most sodas, candies, corn and soy products, the list goes on and on. There are countries that have GMO-free products, because they have banned it, but in the United States you can often only find the GMO option. (Non GMO Project)

The body can take some hits, but if you consume soda or products that contain GMOs all the time, it may be affecting your health.

Pesticide residue is found in 70% of conventional produce sold in the US even after washing it. I know none of us like pests, but our bodies definitely do not like pesticides. One of my keys to health was when I switched over to eating more organic. I always try to EAT AS ORGANIC AS POSSIBLE. I try to buy organic any chance I get. I know that it can be very expensive to buy everything organic.

Choosing to eat organic today is not as cost prohibitive as it once was. More and more farmers are choosing to grow organic as consumer demand has risen. As a single mom living in Hawaii, it's not always affordable for us, but it's my goal and this is why it is important to know about... The Dirty Dozen and the Clean 15.

The Dirty Dozen and The Clean 15

Eating organic and more plant-based is a partnership. It benefits our health and our environment. This is why it is important to know about the Dirty Dozen and the Clean 15.

The Dirty Dozen are the top 12 pesticide-laden foods. You want to avoid these if they are not organic.

The Clean 15 are the cleanest (little to no pesticides). They are easier to grow without the use of them. So you can purchase these conventionally and be ok.

Take a look at the list and try to buy at least the Dirty Dozen as organic. These lists are updated regularly every few years, so make sure to find the most updated list online.

THE DIRTY DOZEN:

1. Strawberries
2. Spinach
3. Kale, collards, and mustard greens
4. Nectarines
5. Apples
6. Grapes
7. Bell and hot peppers
8. Cherries
9. Peaches
10. Pears
11. Celery
12. Tomatoes

THE CLEAN FIFTEEN:

1. Avocado
2. Sweet corn*
3. Pineapple
4. Onions
5. Papaya*
6. Sweet peas (frozen)
7. Asparagus
8. Honeydew melon

---

* Some sweet corn and papaya are often grown from GMO seeds, so I still buy these organic.

9. Kiwi
10. Cabbage
11. Mushrooms
12. Cantaloupe
13. Mangoes
14. Watermelon
15. Sweet potatoes
    (Group)

On Having Your Cake, and Eating it too!

Okay, so with this new-found knowledge—what are we supposed to do? Change everything out? Well that's a process, and let's not forget that divorcing your diet is about the health of your body and mind through food. So, how can food make us feel better? Right now, I want you to remember the feeling that some of your favorite childhood foods gave you. The excitement as you dug into a plate of nachos with friends or sipping fruit smoothies on a warm summer morning. Maybe it was Mom's chili on a fall evening. Now that we know all this great information about food, it's time to take those tried and true classics and make them better so that you're emotionally connected. Both better tasting and better for you.

I am not making a case to be vegan like me, but to be plant-centric, replace a lot of what you eat with simpler plant-based versions of the original. It may not be your grandma's original recipe, but it will hit those A-HAs, that only your favorites can. You can make it with better ingredients that don't cause disease to our planet, animals, or your body. We are adaptable beings and your taste buds will change to craving that vegan ranch over store bought ranch dressing, just give it time and learn how to get it to as close to the original as possible.

On Childhood Favorites

Don't break up with your childhood faves, just make them healthier. I saw a video on Instagram that was called World's Best Tuna Fish Sandwich. As the girl makes the tuna, she says this is the recipe her mom made as a kid, and she says she didn't know why but it's the best. I know why... our brain has chemicals that get released when we eat certain foods, especially ones from our childhood or heritage. This is why you think your recipe is the best. So what if we made it plant-based, or more plant-based, and still had those same chemical levels drop, but not have the bloat, tiredness, and autoimmune symptoms?

I eat all my childhood favorites in a variety of ways. My mom drank tea every morning, Lipton with sugar and 2% milk. I drink a similar tea and use organic black tea with maple syrup or organic sugar and almond milk. This vegan version does the same for my soul, that the original did, just without any of the adverse reactions.

Same with my chili, burritos, sandwiches, and breakfast scrambles, I created a vegan version of everything I ate regularly and it changed my health. I had to learn more and more about ingredients, so I was giving myself all the essential ingredients.

On Eating Out

Eating out at regular restaurants kills me. They normally don't have anything vegan on the menu. I have to remove things or create something and hope the servers write it down correctly. It's the worst, because you are never accidentally served vegan food. There are added animal products in everything and it keeps your body in an inflammatory response. The side of broccoli is covered in cheese. The asparagus is cooked with bacon and butter. The potatoes are cooked in butter and milk. The salads have cheese or meat, and many times the dressings have it too. It can feel impossible at first, but the trick is finding restaurants that are vegan or have vegan menus.

I talked about the muffins in the beginning of this chapter, and just to hit it home, let's compare some more foods. Your body is a complete process and you don't have to understand it. But it does need to break down and separate the nutrients in what you're eating. Think of each ingredient as a puzzle piece. We all could put together a 10 piece puzzle quicker than a 45 piece puzzle. Think about what you are eating.

Fast Food Chicken Sandwich vs. Oyster Mushroom Sandwich

Let's take a look at two sandwiches which may look similar when laid out in front of you, but when you take a closer look at the ingredients you can see that that is the furthest thing from the truth.

FAST FOOD CHAIN Chicken Sandwich

Chicken Sandwich Chicken Filet: chicken containing up to 31% of water, mild seasoning [modified corn starch, monosodium glutamate, salt, dried onion, dried garlic, dried celery, spices (paprika), natural flavor, lactic acid and polysorbate 80], seasoning (modified corn starch, salt, flavor, monosodium glutamate, hydrolyzed dark chicken meat, maltodextrin, partially hydrogenated soybean oil), isolated soy protein (isolated soy protein, modified potato starch, corn starch, carrageenan with less than 2% lecithin), sodium phosphates, and stabilizers (mono and diglycerides, maltodextrin, and sodium phosphate). contains: soy, milk, MSG poultry batter: enriched bleached wheat flour (enriched with niacin, reduced iron, thiamine, mononitrate, riboflavin, folic acid), salt, spack [enriched bleached wheat flour (enriched with niacin, reduced iron, thiamine, mononitrate, riboflavin, folic acid), salt, sugar, fd&c yellow #5 (may also contain yellow #6, red #40, red #3, grape color extract, blue #1, blue #2, beet color extract, annatto extract and/or turmeric extract), spices, dried whole eggs, nonfat dried milk, leavening (sodium bicarbonate and/or sodium aluminum sulfate), microcrystalline cellulose, natural flavor (all flavor ingredients 6 contained in this flavor are approved for use in a regulation of food and drug administration or are listed as generally recognized as safe on a reliable published industry association list. This product also contains corn syrup solids). Contains: wheat, egg, milk and yellow #5 & #6, red #3 and #40, blue #1 and blue #2. flour: bleached wheat flour, malted barley. contains: wheat diamond shaped roll: enriched flour (wheat flour, niacin, reduced iron, ascorbic acid added as a dough conditioner, thiamine mononitrate, riboflavin, folic acid, enzyme), water, yellow corn meal, fructose, salt, gums arabicguar, wheat flour, enzymes, soybean oil, yeast, dough conditioner (mono & diglycerides, wheat flour, malted barley flour, guar gum, datem, dextrose, ascorbic acid, lcysteine, enzymes), malt powder, yeast, enzymes. contains wheat, soy delta sauce: soybean oil, water, mustard (water, vinegar, mustard seed, salt, turmeric, paprika, spices), dill relish (diced pickles, water, salt, vinegar, xanthan gum, sodium benzoate and potassium sorbate (preservatives), natural flavors), food starch modified, creole mustard (water, distilled vinegar, mustard seed, salt, xanthan gum), distilled vinegar, sugar, tomato paste, seasoning (maltodextrin, salt, buttermilk powder, whey powder, monosodium glutamate, lactic acid, citric acid, garlic powder, onion powder, parsley, xanthan gum, soybean oil, spices, artificial flavor), egg yolks, contains less than 2% of each: chipotle peppers, salt, oleoresin paprika, natural flavor, oleoresin capsicum, high fructose corn syrup, corn syrup, cayenne pepper, lemon juice concentrate, molasses, caramel color, garlic*, spices, tamarind, onion*, paprika, partially hydrogenated soybean oil, garlic, monosodium glutamate, ground chipotle peppers, xanthan gum, potassium sorbate and sodium benzoate (preservatives), extractives of paprika, calcium disodium EDTA to protect flavor. *dehydrated. Contains egg, milk, soy, MSG leaf lettuce, tomato slices.

Homemade Fried Oyster Mushroom Sandwich

Fresh French bread rolls, flour, sourdough starter (yeast), water, salt.

Batter—almond milk (almonds, water salt) flour, salt, pepper, avocado oil for frying, oyster mushrooms.

Chipotle vegenaise (expeller-pressed canola oil, filtered water, chipotle chili paste (water, chipotle chiles), garlic, brown rice syrup, white wine vinegar, pea protein, sea salt, mustard flour, natural smoke flavor, lemon juice concentrate, xanthan gum, paprika extract).

Lettuce, tomato.

DELIVERY CHAIN Pizza vs. Organic Vegan Pizza

Let's do another comparison. A popular pizza compared to one made healthfully, even though it is found in the freezer section.

Meaty with Marinara

Crust (enriched flour (bleached wheat flour, malted barley flour, niacin, ferrous sulfate, thiamine mononitrate, riboflavin, folic acid), water, yeast, soybean oil. Contains 2% or less of: salt, vital wheat gluten, datem, sugar, enzymes, ascorbic acid, sucralose), pizza cheese (part skim mozzarella cheese (pasteurized milk and skim milk, cheese cultures, salt, enzymes), sugar cane fiber (added to prevent clumping), modified food starch, potassium chloride, natural flavors, rosemary extract (to protect flavor)), pepperoni (pork, beef, salt, contains 2% or less of: spices, dextrose, lactic acid starter culture, extractives of paprika, extractives of rosemary, sodium nitrite), ham (ham, cured with: water, salt, sodium lactate, sugar, sodium phosphates, sodium diacetate, sodium erythorbate, sodium nitrite), seasoned beef (beef, water, salt, tomato paste, natural flavors, dextrose, dehydrated onion, spice), seasoned pork (pork, water, salt, spices, sugar, autolyzed yeast extract, corn syrup solids, natural flavor), Italian sausage (pork, seasoning (spices, paprika, sugar, garlic powder, salt, spice extractives), water, salt), toasted parmesan cheese (pasteurized milk, cheese culture, salt, enzymes), marinara dipping sauce (tomato paste, water, sugar, salt, garlic powder, spices, and citric acid). contains wheat, milk.

Frozen Vegan Supreme

Organic unbleached wheat flour, filtered water, organic tomato purée, organic vegan mozzarella-style cheese (filtered water, organic potato starch, organic coconut oil, sea salt, organic ground sunflower kernels, natural flavoring, organic fruit and vegetable concentrate [organic carrot, organic pumpkin and organic apple]), organic onions, organic mushrooms, organic extra virgin olive oil, olives, organic tomatoes, soy cheese—mozzarella type (filtered water, organic expeller pressed soybean oil, organic soy-milk powder, natural flavors, inulin [chicory root extract], agar agar, sea salt, organic soy protein, lactic acid), organic bell peppers, organic agave syrup, organic tofu (filtered water, organic soybeans, magnesium chloride), organic wheat gluten, organic cooked cannellini beans, sea salt, expeller pressed high oleic safflower and/or sunflower oil, organic garbanzo bean flour, organic quinoa, organic celery, organic carrots, organic long-grain red rice, tapioca starch, gluten-free oats, organic garlic, organic green lentils, paprika, organic cane sugar, organic potatoes, organic rice flour, spices, mustard powder, organic flax seed meal, yeast, nutritional yeast, black pepper, organic beet root powder, hickory smoke flavor, organic potato flour, organic rice bran extract.

Even though the vegan pizza still has a lot of ingredients, they are still organic and I can still read them and tell you what they are.

An even healthier option would be to make it at home, using the following ingredients—flour, water, yeast, salt, canned Italian tomatoes, red wine, salt, maple syrup, cashews, water, salt, and any toppings you want.

Just remember everyone is selling you something, today in my Instagram ads, a famous actor was selling me health, in a drink that has everything in it for health. Once again, not looking at what you have or need to get to a balanced place so you feel healthy. There was another ad for a 90-day plan that would get me abs following their diet. There are so many diets out there, and as I research more and more, the algorithms of the tech gods now advertise every diet or reason I don't have health and what I need to do to get it. Eat raw? Paleo? Blood sugar? Eat for specific symptoms? Liver cleanse? Take these, avoid those, but what after that? When I'm left to my own devices.

Don't break up with your childhood faves, just make them healthier.

Chapter 4

HOW I EAT AND THINK

My Evolution with Food and Why You Need One

I eat vegan and try to remember what was taught in Kindergarten "You are what you eat," and guess what? It's true. Food is energy and your food is either giving you energy or robbing it from you. None of the foods I eat come from animals, and I don't notice anything missing. I don't believe everyone should be vegan, but I do think everyone should be more vegan-ish.

I have spent a lot of time divorcing different diets and really figuring out what works for me. What worked for me 5 or 10 years ago won't work for me today, so I have started to listen to my body. For example, even though I'm vegan, I don't really eat much soy. As delicious of a meat replacement as it can be, it causes inflammation in my body, and I always wake up with my eyes feeling puffy and tired the next day. So what do I do? I have found other options that work awesome FOR ME, and yes, sometimes I eat soy, because a crumble of tempeh on a salad is delicious and so much healthier than bacon.

Over the years, I have learned—and continue to learn—how to nourish my body based on its daily needs. I do this by making recipes to support my hormones, lower my stress-levels, or increase my energy... it depends on the day. I have found that everyone is unique, so finding what works for each of us and really getting to know our own bodies is a vast challenge, even more so, an immense life-changer. Start by discovering what foods make you simply feel energized and alive. This will increase your energy and overall well-being, and perhaps even prolong your life.

I realized that I should know my body better than anyone, even my doctor. This is something that no one would have told me as a child. It has taken me a long time to discover that I even have the capability of knowing my body on such a level, and all it took was beginning to listen to it. I don't hold the only keys to health, but I do have a keychain of experiences that I want to share to assist in the process of incorporating health, self-love, and wellness into lives. Here are the habits I try to follow in life that help me become the best recipe for a healthy Hollan.

Nourish Yourself

As I talked about before, I eat a lot of the foods I grew up eating, just vegan versions. There are other recipes I have and add to the arsenal, but I eat for my taste buds and body.

I normally start with coffee, it's always organic and I use a French press at home. I add organic sugar or maple syrup and almond or oat milk to it. This is how I had my coffee before, it was just non-organic conventional coffee, sugar, and half and half. I try to drink water before and after my coffee so that whatever goes into my gut from the coffee is diluted. Next, I normally wait an hour and I have a smoothie, protein shake, overnight oats, or avocado toast for breakfast. I try to wait until I am hungry, and that's normally after I work out. By doing this I have learned the difference between hungry and starving.

For lunch, I have a salad or leftovers, and this tends to be my heaviest meal. I try to include lots of leafy greens, some sort of carb (like sweet potato or rice), carrots, cucumbers, and top it off with my homemade dilly ranch dressing.

Later on in the day, I will either have a smoothie or fruit for a snack. If I'm going to yoga or the beach I pack my smoothies in reusable mason jars so they won't spill. They are a perfect sweet and filling treat.

At the end of the day I often have a pasta or potato focused meal for dinner. For dessert I always eat my cheat cookie dough. It's made with almond butter, maple syrup, oats, and chips and it satisfies my sweet tooth. I find maple syrup doesn't spike my sugar as much and the fat from nut butters helps to fill me up.

What I cook also has to taste good, so my kids, Jaden, Kalia, and Lilah, will actually want to eat it. We aren't just eating raw kale over here! As a mom I feel responsibility for them, with this knowledge of which foods are best to keep your body in health. However, they are kids and want all the foods. When they were younger, I would create whatever they wanted, but I would veganize it. They could eat what they wanted on their own (this was hard for me and it still is). They are older now and have to make their own choices. They all know that food affects their health and come back to me when they aren't feeling good. Teach your kids about health whenever you have the opportunity. Kids don't like to hear it, but they do absorb it and can have a better idea about food than you did. Cooking for kids is what taught me diversity in my cooking and I learned how to make anything they wanted vegan.

My Usual Meals or Salads

I do a lot of salads, normally with a nut-based dressing so it fills me. I eat wheat, and have avocado, and vegan sausage sandwiches. I make enchiladas and tacos, and change up the fillings. I make pasta and homemade sauce. I do scrambles in the morning with cauliflower or vegan eggs like Just Eggs™. I make French toast and pancakes. I guess that almost anything you eat, I eat, but vegan.

In the recipes section you will see all the different recipes I make. My food style goes from "ghetto gourmet" as my clients Rocky and Damon Dash call it, and can go all the way to cleansing raw foods. I cook and eat what foods I think will support my body and sometimes I still cook and have periods of only choosing comfort foods.

When I do have a period of eating only for comfort and start to feel less energetic or more irritable I normally will just add a smoothie or salad to my mix to start getting back on track.

A Smoothie or a Salad a Day Gives You Energy

I want you to add one fresh smoothie a day or replace one meal with a salad.

You can have whatever else you like to eat.

I will give you a few smoothie recipes and a few salad recipes, or you can make your own.

You can have a different one every day or stick to the one you love. I just want you to add a smoothie or a salad to how you normally eat and see how you feel.

I also find that both of these meals give me energy. This is a good way to measure your energy after these meals compared to your other meals. This normally reminds me of what good food does and makes me crave healthier foods over comfort foods.

I have had years of laziness where I wasn't working out consistently and where my eating habits led to me choosing foods that were super easy or on taste alone. Then, when I made the switch to choose foods that actually feed my health, it was the difference between vitality and not. Think of a house plant that is dying, leaves withering away, and then you just give it water and the plant perks up, but as soon as you fertilize the plant with what it needs, the plant has a different energy and health. You're a plant and you've been watered with foods that have very little nutrition. Providing yourself with the water, nutrients, and attention your body needs and deserves will give you so many benefits. Our habits don't define us, but they do help us. You can choose habits that pull you out of health or habits that give you vitality. Just like a houseplant, you will notice the change of energy. Like houseplants, you can live on very little and stay in survival mode, withering away, or you can tend to yourself, even a little bit more every day, grow new leaves, and look and feel better.

I try to remember that I am the only one in charge of checking in with me and choosing health. You must hold yourself accountable and make the best choices with your own knowledge. I went through every diet to see there wasn't one that would sustain me.

Going more vegan or plant-based allows you the opportunity to learn more about your health through food and new ingredients than any other diet. Fruits and vegetables are nutrient-dense and full of beneficial fiber, vitamins, and minerals. A diet consisting of grains, fruit, nuts, seeds, and vegetables has been shown to dramatically improve your health. There's only one way to find out, GIVE IT A TRY.

The Case for Soup

For centuries, soup has been recommended when you are sick because soups are full of nutrient-dense vegetables that are slow-cooked, so that these ingredients retain their nutrition, are easy to digest, and are yummy to our palate. Here are reasons why I think soup should be a staple at your dinner table and not just for when you're sick. Soup can help you lose weight. The high water and fiber contents from vegetables added to the soup keeps you satiated in a healthy and hydrating way. Have a bowl of soup for dinner, and you won't overeat. It makes for a hearty meal by itself and provides satiety with fewer calories than most other regular meals. In short, the soup will keep you feeling fuller for longer, make your tummy happy, and can keep your blood sugar levels stable. Unless your soup is made with heavy cream, most recipes include fibrous vegetables, beans, and lentils, which all help with healthy digestion. For those of you who find it hard to eat 7–8 servings of vegetables a day, making a pot of soup to reheat and eat throughout the week is the solution. The slow-cooking method used for soup ensures that it retains the vitamins and minerals of the cooked vegetables since you also consume the broth. Whether you are making a soup with lentils or beans or just with vegetables, you get a full array of nutrients in that delicious broth. Also, some nutrients like beta carotene from carrots and lycopene from tomatoes, are better absorbed by the body when food is cooked rather than when eaten raw. Besides these benefits of soups, the thing I love the most about them is that they're so versatile. You can play around with ingredients to create a warming bowl of goodness with any ingredients at hand. Making soup is also affordable, and since you can use whatever you have, it helps create less food waste!

Hydrating Myself

I am not good at drinking water naturally. I always feel better when I am drinking water and here is how I come back to it when I need to remind myself of how healthy water is for every function of the body.

If you are someone who drinks plenty of water a day, keep it up and carry on. I am not that somebody. I want to be. I am not that naturally thirsty of a person. There is no denying that when I'm on my water game I see so many changes in my skin, glow, and overall health. Water is essential to resetting your body. So, follow the steps below to add more water to your life. The benefits for hydrating yourself with water are amazing.

Just a reminder, water helps...

- Maximize physical performance
- Boost energy levels and brain activity
- Treat headaches

- Help with constipation and kidney stones
- Prevent hangovers
- Help with weight loss
- Balance the body's pH level
- Create clearer skin

I believe that any change you make that is better than the day before is progress. I found various sources of information on the amount of water we need each day. Ask yourself the following questions...

- How many ounces of water do you drink a day?
- How many ounces of other liquids do you drink a day?
- What is your goal physically?
- What exercise level do you fall into?

1 = Nothing, 10 = Marathon Runner

Total the number of liquid ounces you drink in a day, and switch over to all water, and omit the other beverages. Not ready for that yet? Try this... Drink that total number of fluid ounces in water before you have anything else to drink throughout the day.

Let's say you drink 24 ounces of water, 12 ounces of coffee, and 12 ounces soda a day for a total of 48 ounces a day. I want you to start by upping your water intake to 48 ounces daily.

Are you training for a marathon or have a physically demanding job? Your body needs lots of water, at least 100 ounces a day! Start to track your water, and see where you feel your best.

AGAIN, I believe that any change you make that is better than the day before is progress. I just want you to grow. I don't need you to be perfect. I just need you to see where you can better support yourself, and hydrating with water is where you start.

I use a Berkey™ water filter at my house. I love the water. I do not recommend plastic water bottles. I find its most accessible to have your own reusable water bottle with you all the time. If you forget it, splurge and buy water in a glass bottle. It's better for you, and the planet.

Here are the steps I follow when I find I'm not watering myself...

- I drink 16 ounces of water as soon as I rise. It's a great way to start the day, and give my body what it needs after rest—clear, clean water. Is there anything more cleansing? (If you drink coffee, this is crucial. You do not want the first thing your body gets to be acidic coffee.)
- Every time I use the bathroom, I drink water. Replace what goes out.
- Every time I finish a glass I refill it and leave it on the counter. I am more likely to drink it if it's there and ready.
- I drink out of my favorite crystal water bottle. I love drinking out of it. I always think happy, healing thoughts when I look at it. I also love my Hydro Flask. It keeps my ice water cold in the summer, and warm water toasty in the winter. Just get a water bottle you love. Fill it up and bring it with you everywhere. I mean everywhere. You are more likely to drink water if it is with you.
- I add fruit to the water to make it fun, colorful, and lightly flavored. Go crazy! I love mint and cucumber, watermelon and blueberry, or pineapple and mango.

Movement and Exercise

Next I exercise. I move my body. I am lucky enough to live somewhere that forces me to be active, but I still workout. Not only does it help the body and strengthen it, it also helps with your mental health. Any time I feel depressed and lackluster, I move my body more. Exercise improves your overall health and helps boost your immune system. Some studies show that "moderate to intense" exercise may cut down the number of colds you get. Do something you love. Go for a walk, go to yoga, Pilates, a run, or anything you like, just start moving.

I want you to move. Even just for today. I don't care if it's a 5-minute walk you wouldn't typically take, or if you start training for that marathon. Just move today more than you usually would. I have done Pilates and yoga 2–3 days a week for many years. It has become habitual. You know what happens to me when I don't go for a week or two? I start feeling lethargic, moody, and anxiety starts settling in. Every time I go back to it, I notice I have energy, my mood stabilizes, and I have no more fear. I do know for sure that our bodies were meant for more than sitting. Bodies actually thrive if you give them just a little love and attention. I work out for my body, my mind, and to have my body maintain its vitality as I age. I am stronger and more flexible now than I was in my 30s. I have more mobility than I did in my 20s. I attribute this all to investing a little time and making it non-negotiable in my life to move my body.

There is no right or wrong workout, whether you are a walker, runner, gym rat, sports lover, yogi, or love Pilates, just do something. Push yourself more. Make goals, keep them.

In a journal or on a piece of paper, write what you did, give yourself a high five and make a commitment to add some sort of movement into your life. Give yourself a goal. Write a sentence about how you will move toward it.

Then add, Here is my list:

- I went on a walk today! 30 minutes, 2 miles, HIGH 5!
- I would like to add this to my life 2 × week.
- I will wake up at 6 a.m. Tuesdays and Thursdays and walk.
- By the end of the year, I would like to progress to 3 days a week.

Promise yourself. Follow through, and that's it.

Sleep Well

After a full day, rest is so important and underrated. It sets your hormones processes for the day. It's your body's reset. Research has shown that a good night's sleep helps build your immune cells, also known as T-cells. The amount of sleep you need varies from person to person. You want to wake up feeling well-rested. That could be 6, 8, or even 10 hours. Check-in with yourself and see where you feel your best, and then sleep accordingly. I once read an article that suggested humans sleep in increments of 1½ hour loops. A lot of times we wake up naturally at the end of a cycle, to go to the bathroom, or just wake up. The researcher claimed that when we go back to bed, and we are unable to go through another 1½ hour cycle, we will wake up groggy in the middle of it. So before you give yourself 30 minutes more in the morning, see if you can wake up naturally by staying up, or go back to bed if you have 90 minutes to complete it. Experiment with this, because this step has changed my life. I have more energy throughout my day, and no crash and burn in the middle of it. Overall, I feel healthier whenever I am following this routine. (NEIL-SHERWOOD)

Manifest

Right now is a good time to put in the work on creating the life we want. One of my favorite books, *Breaking the Habit of Being Yourself* by Joe Dispenza, teaches ways to become more than you thought you could be. It calms the nervous system and forces you to look at what past heartache, traumas, and beliefs are holding you back. I don't know what speaks to you, but, whatever you believe, study it and educate yourself in being better. I have always been a big believer in manifesting and creating the life you want. In the book *You Squared* this quote changed me, "The only doubts you should have are your limits." How many of you have a bigger dream than what you are living? Start aligning with that part of yourself. I believe it is our inner voice guiding us.

Talk to Someone

It can feel impossible to make these changes for your body, mind, and health without having someone to talk to. Just like leaving an ex, you need support to make sure you are doing what's best for you. Whether this is someone who wants to work with you so that you have an accountability buddy, or just someone to talk to on those days when you would really rather swallow those feelings with food.

What is important is making sure that the people we surround ourselves with aren't toxic. When you are in a toxic friendship or relationship, your body goes into a fight or flight mode, which comprises your immune system and body. Chemicals are released into your bloodstream, which wreak havoc on your system. Remember, humans are not supposed to be in a trauma trigger most of the time.

The top five people around you influence the way you live, so always choose wisely, but especially when your health is on the line. We are supposed to be a community, lifting each other up, feeling filled by each other, not drained.

You see, divorcing your diet is really about divorcing so many things in your life and learning what you really need to support you. The relationship you have with your health is about how you take care of yourself in so many ways, not just with food. I wouldn't be here writing this book today if I didn't look at all areas of my life that needed change, continuously, and unfortunately still have to. No one is coming to save you and make the changes you need to make. You are the knight in shining armor you have been waiting for.

Now back to food, ready to learn how to transform those recipes you love? A note on cooking for yourself. I meet so many people that tell me they can't cook. I think everyone should learn how to. When you cook for yourself, you get to make foods that are perfect for your taste buds. Just the right amount of salty, spicy, and sweet that you like. Being in a kitchen is a practical art. Meaning the more you practice the better you get. I am a very fast chef, but it wasn't that way naturally, it's because I have done it for so many years and have practiced. So If you don't cook, here is your invitation from me, to enter the kitchen, it's never too late to learn how to cook. In the back of the book, there are resources for my favorite tools in the kitchen that make prep and cooking that much easier.

A Note on Cleansing/Resetting

By giving your body a break from foods that cause inflammation you can unleash your own superpowers. I believe there is an evolution with the response your body has to different foods, and that, if we give our bodies breaks from those foods for a certain amount of time, our bodies reset. They start to work for us and not against us. Our cells are capable of cleansing and cleaning out our bodies if we give them time and space to reset from digesting the same foods, day after day. At times I need to reset. I normally know this because I have a lack of energy or my body is giving me symptoms, like headaches, itchy skin, or pain.

I believe if we look at it from a natural state, everything has seasons. There is very little that is available to us year round without modern society. Certain foods definitely have longer seasons than others. I give up certain foods for weeks or months out of the year. Here are some examples of foods I take breaks from:

- Gluten
- Grains
- Beans
- Fruit
- Sugar
- All potatoes

Even though I give up fruit for small periods, I also believe in the power of FRUIT. I think it is God's gift of perfect food. It is sweet, yummy, and pre-packaged. I do give myself weeks at a time throughout the year where I do not have sugar, including fruit, but that means that when I come back to it, it is better than ever!

This is the trick to how I stay healthy and have balance with eating foods I love most of the time. I JUST RESET.

I would actually call it a rest reset, where I give my body a rest from ingredients I know my body has issues with when I am eating too much of a certain ingredient, like too much sugar, too much gluten, or too many carbs. There can be too much of a good thing. So I give my body a rest from these ingredients and give it time to heal. I literally base it off of how I'm feeling. None of this should be long term, and it really is just simplifying what you're eating.

Reset 1 - Vegan, No Coffee

I start with the basics, which is cutting out coffee. If I had a soul mate in my life, it would be coffee. This is the hardest thing I do, but it gives me the opportunity to nourish and cleanse my body with clear liquids. I give myself a break from the acid and caffeine. I always feel better. But I always go back to it because it is one of the loves of my life. There is nothing I enjoy more than a warm cup of coffee, sitting in my backyard, and watching the sunrise over the mountains in Kauai.

Reset 2- Vegan, No Coffee, No Gluten

I go gluten-free. I still eat bread, just gluten-free options. Gluten is the protein found in wheat, barley, rye, spelt, and other products. It is indigestible, like many components of food we eat. This isn't really a problem, unless you start changing the amount of gluten naturally found in these products, or are eating an abundance of gluten. I have found that sometimes my body reacts to wheat/gluten and other times has no issues. This has made me have a love/hate relationship with it, as I never know how it will affect me.

For the most part, I try to vary my grains and only eat gluten in moderation. If I feel it is not working for me, I give my system a chance to recover by not eating it at all. I have found that when I have been gluten-free and eat too many gluten-free replacements (breads, tortillas, etc.) I start to have the same issues as if I were eating gluten. Over the years, I have attributed this to what I call the "abundance factor." When I eat an abundance of processed foods (breads, crackers, chips, cookies) my body doesn't handle it well, and it starts giving me cues (disease and symptoms), so I adjust where I can.

A small percentage of the population have a disease related to gluten called celiac disease. For persons with celiac disease, even a pinch of gluten is extremely toxic to their system, and will create symptoms and problems affecting their body's ability to process and use the nutrients from foods. If you suspect gluten is wreaking havoc on your system, there is an easy test you can perform—stop eating it and see how you feel. Once again, it's about listening to your body. That's exactly what we are going to do. Give up gluten for a week and see how you feel.

Reset 3- Vegan, No Coffee, No Gluten, No Grains

After a few days of eliminating gluten, I switch it up and go grain free. I know that this can seem extreme, but remember that, in nature, there would be seasons where we don't have access to these grains all the time, and our bodies may need breaks from it. Instead of a base of rice or quinoa, I use starchy mashed potatoes. I do smoothies 2 times a day during this. I eat a lot of salads and soups that are filling and full of whole food ingredients.

Reset 4– Vegan, No Coffee, No Gluten, No Grains, No Sugar, No Fruit

After a few days of grain free, I then cut out fruit and sugar. So, it's even more extreme, but it's actually simple. In society, we see eating this way as extreme, but if we were in the wild in winter, this would be normal. This will give my body time to rest from regulating my sugar. I stay on this part of the reset until I feel done, maybe a few days, maybe a week. It just depends on where I am health wise and my goals.

You can just do any of these resets or you can follow the evoulution of all of them. If you're hungry, eat more, there are no rules.

To give you a better idea of what this looks like, here is a sample 3-day menu from each one of the phases.

Reset 1 - Vegan, No Coffee
(A beginner reset)

Day 1:
Breakfast
- Smoothie of choice

10 a.m. Snack
- Apple with almond butter

Lunch
- Avocado sandwich

4 p.m. Snack
- Crackers and hummus

Dinner
- BBQ cauliflower, with rice, and green beans

Dessert
- Protein shake

Day 2:
Breakfast
- Fruit salad

10 a.m. Snack
- Protein shake

Lunch
- Leftover cauliflower and rice

4 p.m. Snack
- Protein ball/bar

Dinner
- Mac and cheese please

Dessert
- Riced Krispy treat

Day 3:
Breakfast
- Cauliflower scramble

10 a.m. Snack
- Blueberries

Lunch
- BLT

4 p.m. Snack
- Protein shake

Dinner
- Lentil soup with bread and a side salad

Dessert
- Store bought vegan ice cream

Reset 2 – Vegan, No Coffee, No Gluten
(Checking in on yourself)

Day 1:
Breakfast
- Almond butter banana toast

10 a.m. Snack
- Protein shake (chocolate)

Lunch
- Garden salad with ranch

4 p.m. Snack
- Celery with almond butter and raisins

Dinner
- Cream of mushroom or cauliflower soup with gluten-free crackers and a side salad

Dessert
- Brownies (gfree)

Day 2:
Breakfast
- Overnight blueberry oats

10 a.m. Snack
- Protein ball/bar

Lunch
- Leftover soup

4 p.m. Snack
- Apple with almond butter

Dinner
- Gluten free enchiladas

Dessert
- Fresh fruit cocktail

Day 3:

Breakfast
- Avocado toast

10 a.m. Snack
- Smoothie

Lunch
- Leftover enchilada

4 p.m. Snack
- Crackers and hummus

Dinner
- Eggplant no parmesan and a side salad

Dessert
- Dried apricots with chocolate chips

Reset 3 - Vegan, No Coffee, No Gluten, No Grain
(Back to Simple)

Day 1:

Breakfast
- Smoothie

Lunch
- Garbanzo bean tuna lettuce cups

Dinner
- Sweet potato Leek stew

Dessert
- Protein shake

Day 2:

Breakfast
- Chia pudding with fruit

<u>Lunch</u>
- Leftover soup

<u>Dinner</u>
- Zucchini noodles with nutritional yeast

<u>Dessert</u>
- Protein shake

Day 3:
<u>Breakfast</u>
- Sweet potato with vegan butter

<u>Lunch</u>
- Leftover noodles

<u>Dinner</u>
- Caesar salad with sweet potato

<u>Dessert</u>
- Protein shake

Reset 4 - Vegan, No Coffee, No Gluten, No Grains, No Sugar, No Fruit
(No Way to Live)

Day 1:
<u>Breakfast</u>
- Protein shake

<u>Lunch</u>
- Chili quesadilla

<u>Dinner</u>
- Kale salad with sweet potato

Day 2:

Breakfast

- Protein shake

Lunch

- Leftover potato and kale

Dinner

- Eggplant no parmesan, and a side salad

Day 3:

Breakfast

- Protein shake

Lunch

- Leftover eggplant

Dinner

- Cream of mushroom soup

There are no rules to snacking, just try to have it meet the criteria of what phase you are in. Take note of when you feel your best, and as you move forward maybe eliminate that ingredient (coffee, gluten, grains, or sugar) for a while. I use the check-in tool in chapter 2 when I am resetting. After, I go back to my normal healthy eating with a body more ready and equipped to eat "normal foods."

Once again, I can't stress enough that these resets are no way to live unless you have an allergy or Celiac disease. As we learned in chapter 2, our bodies need a variety of nutrients, vitamins, and minerals. Here's where the body gets a little tricky, because it also needs rest.

Some of these recipes listed are in the Reset section of chapters 6 and 7—Recipes.

I could write a whole book on this, too.

I only do this throughout the year when I feel like my body could use a break or I'm having symptoms or have fallen off my program.

Now, on to the fun part, I'm going to teach you about all the amazing products I love and use daily. I have been testing out all the wonderful plant-based products so you don't have to! There are new products all the time, so if you find your taste buds are different from mine, try different things. Before you read the next chapter, make sure to note where your closest co-op, Whole Foods™, or other natural grocery store (or even natural section in your grocery store). I will also be giving you tips and tricks for eating out, and a list of my personal favorite restaurants. I have scoured the interiors of your kitchens and here is what I recommend you start to replace in your diet. You don't have to give up everything and, really, because you are in a relationship with food for the rest of your life, you can take it slow and just start to make better choices with less ingredients. Remember, small changes over a long period of time creates change.

Going more vegan or plant-based allows you the opportunity to learn more about your health through food and new ingredients than any other diet.

Chapter 5

REPLACEMENT GUIDE

The Reason I Can Still Eat This Way

This is the list of plant-based foods I use to replace ingredients in my recipes. This guide will help you replace products, either all at once or slowly over time as you need them. As I have stated before, the ingredients list is most important and what I want you to look at. I give some brand names I recommend while others are general (for example, "pasta" for "organic pasta") and please, even if it's organic, look at ingredient labels before buying it. I will show you what products I love so that you can start replacing the ones you already have in your fridge. Just a healthier alternative. The transition to a healthier life is about to get more comfortable.

I use many of these ingredients in place of all the old toxic ones in my recipes. I believe that if you just swap out what you eat for plant-based versions that are healthier, you will see a dramatic shift in your body and energy. This is a guide to give you ideas about what you can swap for what.

There are so many wonderful products available these days that if you don't find what I recommend, try something new.

There are times that I have to improvise, but what I've listed are my favorites.

Milks (Sweet and Savory)

What you need to know about non-dairy milk and creamer is that there are so many different types. Some are more like non-fat milk, others closer to 2%, and the creamers are closer to whole milk. It is essential to find one that you love, so you don't go back.

The replacements for milk keep coming, but the most popular are:

- Almond Milk
- Soy Milk
- Cashew Milk
- Oat Milk
- Hemp Milk
- Coconut Milk
- Rice Milk

It is so easy to replace milk in any recipe. If it's vanilla or flavored milk it may not be suitable for your savory dishes. I love it in a smoothie, but vanilla mashed potatoes are not my favorite.

I prefer almond milk for everything. The refrigerated ones are creamier than what you find on the shelf.

My recommended brands:

- Califia Farms™
- Malk Organics™
- Elmhurst Creamery™
- Three Trees™

If you prefer shelf stable:

- Cadia™
- Pacific Foods™

Creamers / Half and Half

New creamers are popping up every day. I find that most of them don't stand up to the original. They aren't as creamy or thick. There are so many on the market and some are creamier than others.

- Soy creamer
- Oat creamer
- Coconut creamer
- Almond creamer
- Stir in creamer

My favorite creamers are oat or almond to replace half and half. My favorite brands:

- So Delicious™
- Laird Superfood™ (stir-in)
- Califia Farms™
- Milkadamia™

Many brands also have flavoring if that's your jam.

Butter and Cream Cheese

I first tried vegan butter 17 years ago when I was at a friend's dinner party, and it was all I could talk about. I loved it more than butter. I made the switch to vegan butter before I was ever vegan. Technically it is marginine, but many are made with healthier oils. Try it and see how you feel. My favorite brands are:

- Earth Balance™
- Miyoko's Creamery™
- Melt Organic™
- Milkadamia™

I always buy their soy-free variety when available and use it in place of anything you would use butter for. The possibilities are endless and the sky's the limit.

For cream cheese, I love the brand Kite Hill™, and the creators of it also own my favorite restaurant in Los Angeles, Crossroads! They have so many different flavors, which are good on top of bagels and also as dips. Vegan cream cheese is great as a substitute in any recipes that call for cream cheese.

Other brands I recommend:

- Violife™
- Follow Your Heart™

Cheeses

When I started eating vegan, there were hardly any vegan cheeses available. I often made my own using cashews. Today there are so many different brands and varieties of vegan cheeses available. They are often made with different ingredients like almonds, cashews, nutritional yeast, soy, and coconut. You can find cheese for sandwiches, nachos, pizza, or for charcuterie boards. There is a cheese replacement for anything you would want to make! I also feel the need to tell you about cashew cheese. It's amazing. I use it all the time to make my sauces creamy or in any cooked dishes. It is so easy to make that I use it more than any store-bought variety. Don't like cashews? You can do the same with macadamia nuts, sunflower seeds, or any nut you like in a cheese form. When it bakes it loses its water and resembles ricotta (recipe in chapter 6).

Here are some of my other personal favorite brands:

- Daiya Cheese™
- Chao™
- Follow Your Heart™
- Violife™

Yogurts

Yogurts can be used for so many different recipes. In many cultures, you will find recipes with yogurt as a base or as a topping. Yogurt contains cultures called probiotics that are great for gut health. It is normally easily digestible, and has enough fat to be filling. You don't need to have the dairy to have all the benefits of yogurt.

Here are some of my personal favorite yogurts:

- Cocoyo™ (raw and sugar-free)
- Kite Hill™
- So Delicious™
- Forager Project™

Sour Cream

Sour cream is the perfect topping to a delicious baked potato. It is also a necessary topping for my favorite chili recipe.

Here are some of my favorite brands:

- Forager Project™
- Tofutti™
- Homemade Cashew Cream

Eggs

A lot of times I use tofu as an egg replacement. Crumbled and firm for a scramble or fried, medium for poaching, and silken for baked goods. However, I am allergic to soy and had to find other replacements. For a scramble I use riced cauliflower, for baking I use the water from garbanzo beans (aquafaba) and the replacements below.

- Cauliflower
- Tofu (poached, fried, or scrambled)
- Aquafaba (garbanzo bean water)

Brands I reccomend:

- Just Egg™
- Bob's Red Mill™
- Follow Your Heart™

Tofu

Tofu is delicious and takes on any flavor it's marinating in.
    I love the brands:

- Wildwood™
- House Foods™

- You want to always buy soy organic as conventional soy is genetically modified.

Meats

There are so many plants and nuts you can use to substitue meat. I tend to try an use whole foods wherever I can however there are brands I recommend that are simple and delish to use as a replacement.

Sausages

- Field Roast™
- Tofurky™
- Beyond Meat™

Burgers

- Beyond Meat™
- Amy's Kitchen™
- Sunshine Burgers™

Chicken

- Beyond Meat™
- Alpha Foods™
- Jack and Annies™

Hot Dogs

- Tofu Pups™
- Field Roast™
- Beyond Meat™

Condiments

What is life without condiments? I for one don't want to know.

Mayo

- Follow Your Heart™
  It is my favorite and the only one I recommend.

Ketchup / Mustard / Relish

- Organic ketchup
- Organic mustard
- Organic relish
- Woodstock Eat Because It's Good!™
- Annie's Homegrown™

Soy Sauce / Teriyaki

- SAN-J™
- Braggs Organic™

Coconut Aminos

- Coconut Secret™
- Braggs Organic™

BBQ Sauce

- Annie's Homegrown™
- Woodstock Eat Beacuse It's Good!™

Pasta Sauce

- Any organic (non-dairy) tomato sauce
- Pesto (no cheese please)
- Organico Bello™
- Raos Homemade since 1896™

Nutritional Yeast

- Bob's Red Mill™
- From the bulk bin from your local co-op

Nut Butter and Jelly

- Organic without added ingredients

Salad Dressings

- Annie's Homegrown™
- Braggs Organics™
- Follow Your Heart™
- Homemade

Hummus and Dips

- Homemade
- Sabra Organic™
- Cedars Organic™
- 365 by Whole Foods Market™
- Safeway Organics™
- Bitchin' Sauce™

Oils and Vinegars

- Olive oil
- Avocado oil
- Sunflower oil
- Balsamic vinegar
- Rice vinegar
- Apple Cider vinegar

Pantry Items

The basic pantry items you should swap.

Pasta

- Montebello™
  Gluten-Free
- Tinkyada™
  Grain-Free
- Banza™

Noodles

- Thai Kitchen™
- Eden Foods™

Rice

- Lundberg™
- Buy bulk when available

Canned Beans

- Westbrae Naturals™
- Eden Foods™
- Cadia™

Dried Beans

- Anything organic
- Buy bulk when available

Soups

- Amy's Kitchen™
- Pacific Naturals™
- Imagine Foods™

- Make your own

Breads

- Make my own when served as a side with lunch or dinner
- Inked Organics™
- Dave's Killer Bread™
- Alvarado Street Bakery™
- Ezekiel™
- Rudi's™

Lots of breads are naturally vegan, but double check they are organic and don't contain added sweeteners.

Bagels / English Muffins

- Dave's Killer Bread™
- Rudi's™
- Ezekiel™

Tortillas (corn or flour)

- La Tortilla Factory™
- Indianlife Foods™
  Gluten and Grain Free
- Siete ™

Check labels, but lots of these are naturally vegan

Taco Shells

- Make your own using organic tortillas
- Garden of Eatin'™
  Mainly vegan, but check labels

Croutons

- Edward and Sons™
- Make your own

Chips/Crackers

- Garden of Eatin'™
- Cabo Chips™
- Kettle Brand™
- Siete™
- Lundberg™
- Simple Mill Crackers™
- Any organic replacement for a cracker you love

Mac n Cheese

- Annie's Homegrown™
- Daiya™
- Homemade

Chocolate Chips

- Enjoy Life™
- Buy bulk non-dairy chocolate when available

Freezer Items

Frozen French Fries

- Buy organic
- Alexia™

Waffles

- Vans™

Burritos

- Amy's Kitchen™
- Alpha Foods™
- Sweet Earth™

Entrees

- Amy's Kitchen™
- Field Roast ™

Pizza

- Amy's Kitchen™
- Daiya™

Appetizers

- Annie's Homegrown™
- Amy's Kitchen™

Frozen Fruit / Veggies

- Organic variety only

I make sure all my frozen fruit and vegetables are organic. You can save money by buying large amounts frozen in bulk at big box stores because freezer life is longer than fresh. Also freeze any fruit before it goes bad to add to your smoothies.

Sweet Treats and Baking Swaps

Ice Cream

- NadaMoo™
- So Delicious™

- Ben and Jerry's™ (non-dairy)
- Homemade

Pudding

- Zen™
- Homemade

Cookies/Bars

- Newmans Own™
- Annie's Homegrown™
- Uncle Eddies™
- Simple Mills Crackers™
- Enjoy Life™
- Homemade brownies
- Homemade cookies

Candy / Chocolate Bars

- Justin's™
- Red Vines™ (made simple)
- Surf Snack™
- Unreal™
- Hu™
- YumEarth™

Marshmallows

- Dandies™
- Trader Joe's™

Whipped Cream

- Soyatoo™
- So Delicious™
- Homemade

Flours

- Change to organic flour, whatever flour you prefer. In my pantry you will find: all purpose, brown rice, and almond flour. I stay away from enriched foods.

I love the brands

- Bob's Red Mill™
- King Arthur Baking Company™

Oats

- Organic rolled oats
- Bob's Red Mill™ (they have a gluten-free variety if you have celiac disease)

Sugar

- Organic cane sugar
- Maple syrup
- Organic brown sugar
- Organic powdered sugar

Baking Soda and Baking Powder

- Bob's Red Mill™
- Organic aluminum-free replacement

Cocoa Powder

- Navitas™

Shortening

- Navitas™
- Spectrum™

Drinks

Caffeine

- Coffee (switch to organic)
- Black teas (switch to organic)
- Yerba mate

Soda and Juice

- Switch to organic
- GT's Living Foods™ Synergy™
- Blue Skies™
- Virgil's™
- Zevia™ (sugar free)

Sparkling Water

- San Pellegrino™

Freshly Squeezed Juice

- Freshly squeezed only please

Herbal Teas

- Peppermint tea
- Sweet rose
- Raspberry Leaf tea
- Chamomile

Wine and Beer

- Switch to organic

Where do I shop?

If you don't have a Whole Foods™ near you, I'll bet there is a health food store somewhere close by. Here in Kauai, we have five small health food stores. I shop at all five, as they all offer different products. I have my main one, but do small shops at the others. My kids eat a lot, so I shop a lot.

We don't have Whole Foods™ here, which is nice as Kauai is quaint and small with smaller businesses. I do enjoy them anytime I travel. I don't know if I would cook if I lived near one because they have so many prepared foods.

In Hawaii, it is very expensive to have food shipped, but if you are on the mainland, a quick Google search will find you an online health food store that delivers. Since Amazon™ bought Whole Foods™, you can have it delivered right to your door.

Farmers markets are another great way to find organic fruits and veggies.

I love when you can get fresh bread along with other products as well. It's a big plus as you are supporting local farmers as well as your body by giving it the freshest food.

Any unprocessed plant food is vegan, this includes fruit, vegetables, nuts, seeds, beans, and legumes.

Packaged Foods

Start by scanning the product's label and packaging. Due to the rise of veganism, in the last few years more and more products are being labeled as vegan. Look for products that say "Suitable for Vegans" or have the "Certified Vegan" logo.

Allergies

Find the allergy information of a product by looking near the very bottom of its ingredient list. If the product contains milk, eggs, or shellfish it will plainly say, "Contains milk, eggs, shellfish." This doesn't work so well for products containing meat, but it will quickly tell you whether or not it's worth reading the whole ingredients list or not.

Read the Ingredients

There are many by-products derived from animals that can cause some confusion at first, for example; *whey powder, casein*, and *modified milk ingredients* are all dairy products. Don't let that scare you! You'll be amazed at how quickly you learn what ingredients to avoid. It's nothing to cry over, you'll learn it all in time!

Avoid products with the following listed in the ingredients:

- Casein
- Whey
- Gelatin
- Eggs
- Cheese
- Red #40

Restaurants

When eating out, I seek out vegan restaurants. Normally, I just Google where I am and vegan restaurants. Yelp helps a lot as well. It will show you vegan places and places with vegan options.

There are websites like Happycow.com that list vegan or vegetarian cafes and options. I travel a lot, and places like Los Angeles, San Francisco, and New York City are vegan heaven. There are all sorts of options like vegan Mexican, sushi, Thai, and Indian food. As well as fancier restaurants, even vegan diners!

Take a peek and see what is near you. If you have a Whole Foods™ near you or a health food store, they usually have hot food items, sandwiches, and a salad bar.

When I eat out at non-vegan restaurants, I will give you some examples of what I may order. At a café, I would order a salad without cheese and possibly add avocado. I would look at what sides I could order and if any look good. I would check the soups and see if any are vegan options (many are).

Sandwiches and Delis

1. Whatever vegan bread you like (most are). I love sourdough or French rolls.
2. If you are at a Whole Foods™ they have vegan mayo.
3. If not, mustard is vegan.
4. I get avocado, tomato, onions, pickles, and lettuces, all vegan.

This is my favorite. Most delis can make something like this.

Mexican Foods

I check if their beans are vegan. I check if their rice is vegan and then I order accordingly. I normally get a burrito with beans, rice, avocado or guacamole, lettuce and onions. Chipotle™

nationwide carries sofritos, which are a delicious soy-based meat replacement.

Pizza

Most of the crusts are vegan. Many places have a gluten-free crust as well.

I am lucky that there are a few places here on Kauai that offer vegan cheese.

So I order pizza how I normally like it. I also sometimes get it with no cheese and order a side of marinara. My favorites toppings are pineapple, spinach, black olives and onions or artichokes, sun dried tomato, black olive, and garlic.

Pasta

For the most part, pasta is vegan, unless it's called egg pasta. Marinara is vegan as well, just tell them to hold the parmesan. Sometimes I order noodles, with olive oil, garlic and salt. It's simple and filling. I normally get a side salad with vinaigrette

Burgers

A lot of burger places have a vegan burger. It amazes me. Look for a burger joint that has a vegan option. They are amazing.

Breakfast

Breakfast is tricky and why I look for vegan places. When in a bind, there is always fresh fruit. Oatmeal if they have non-dairy milk. Hash Browns. Maybe a veggie scramble. See if they have bagels and hummus. Add a tomato and you're in heaven.

Here is a list of my favorite restaurants and cafes when I am traveling for work or pleasure. I am always inspired to be a better cook when I try other chefs' food.

Los Angeles Restaurant Recommendations

- SAGE Bistro, Echo Park, Culver City, and Pasadena
- Araya Thai, Wilshire Beverly Area
- Crossroads, Beverly Hills, Las Vegas, and Calabasas, this is one of my favorite upscale restaurants
- Gracias Madre, Mexican Upscale, Beverly Hills
- Flore, casual, Sunset Silverlake
- Plant, Food and Wine, Venice
- Native Foods, fast casual, delish, all over
- Double Zero, pizza, downtown
- Veggie Grill, love fast casual, all over
- Plant Power, love fast casual, all over
- Cafe Gratitude, Larchmont Area

Los Angeles Restaurant Recommendations

- Whole Foods™, Manhattan Beach Area, Venice
- Erewhon Market™, Venice, Wilshire

San Francisco Market Recommendations

- Vegan Burg, burgers fast casual, Haight Ashbury
- Next Level Burger, burgers fast casual, Potrero Hill
- Vegan Picnic, to-go sandwiches and pastries Marina

- Check for Veggie Grill and Native Foods, as they are expanding to Northern California
- Shizen, vegan sushi, Mission
- Greens, vegetarian upscale dining, Marina
- Gracias Madre, Mexican upscale, Mission
- Plant Power, love fast casual, all over
- Veg Grill, love fast casual, all over

San Francisco Market Recommendations

- Whole Foods™ Market
- Rainbow Foods
- Google search closest whole foods or natural food markets

New York City Restaurant Recommendations

- Cinnamon Snail, casual sandwiches, donuts, wall street, Madison Square
- Blossom Du Jour, casual, multiple locations
- Double Zero, pizza, downtown
- Peace Food café, sit down casual, multiple locations
- Erin McKenna's Bakery, gluten-free vegan bakery
- Planta Queen, sushi
- Beyond Sushi, sushi

New York City Market Recommendations

- Whole Foods™ Market, multiple locations

As I have stated before, it is most important that you start to re-place ingredients in the way you eat, not to eat the way I eat. Use the replacement guide to replace whatever ingredients you use in your recipes with the closest variation. If the recipe calls for oil, choose a high quality organic one. I tend to use olive oil and av-ocado oil. If your recipe calls for butter, use vegan butter. For flour, use organic flour. Milk, use plant milk. Anywhere you can replace, you are less likely to be inflamed. So if you are going to have that steak tonight, have it on vegan mashed potatoes with a vegan salad. Try to make your grandma's lasagna with vegan sausage and cashew cheese. It's all about making meals more sim-ple than the original while still keeping the taste. When you make baked goods try using vegan egg replacement and organic ingre-dients and see if it makes you feel the same way.

So, if you wake up and have coffee with half and half or cow's milk, try to find a replacement and see if you feel better in a week. If you have a turkey sandwich for lunch, what if instead you did vegan mayo mustard and sub avocado for the meat and cheese.

What if you took your soup recipes and used veggie broth and replaced the meat with a vegetable? When I started replacing my favorite foods with healthier organic ingredients, I started notic-ing changes. Certain foods that made me feel good emotionally but left my body feeling tired and bloated, in their healthier form they made my body feel good and still hit those emotional needs. The more I did, the more my body healed. I don't know what it will be like for you, but this changed my life, without changing my daily life and food wants. If you love Oreos, try Newman O's and see if you still feel bad. Quality matters. We live in a society where we say fruit has too much sugar and don't eat from the abundance that nature offers, and instead raise animals out of their natural environments to feed us.

Chapter 6

RECIPES

Why I Love Cooking My Own Food
Your Rebound Playlist

Mint Chip Smoothie

I Heart Blueberries Smoothie

Monkey Milk

Mixed Berry Smoothie

PB and Strawberry Smoothie

Coco Whipped Cream

Yummy Yummy Fruit Salad

Banana Pancakes

Blueberry Muffins

Croissants

English Breakfast (Full Menu)

Bagel Sandwich

Avocado Toast

BLT Please

Cream of Mushroom Soup

Caesar Salad

Taco Salad

Ranched Salad

Cauliflower Quiche

Jackfruit Nachos

Pasta Marinara

Enchiladas

Cashew Cheese

Mac and Cheese Please

BBQ Cauli—Power

Brownies

Churros with Chocolate Dip

Riced Crispy Treats should be moved up and listed directly under Churros with Chocolate Dip

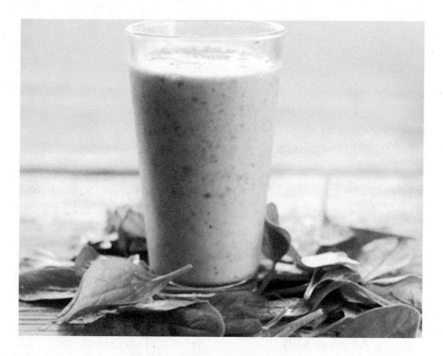

Mint Chip Smoothie

What I love about this smoothie is that it's a way to get spinach, fresh mint, and bananas in my body first thing in the morning. Even though it is nutritious it is delish!

Serves 1 (16 oz.) smoothie
Prep Time: 5 Minutes
GF

Ingredients:
- ½ cup of fresh spinach
- 2 frozen bananas
- ¼ bunch fresh mint
- 1 cup almond milk
- 2 ice cubes
- 2 tbsp. chocolate chips or cacao nibs

In a blender add everything except for the chocolate chips. Start blending on low and gradually bring it up to high until everything is pulverized. Bring back to low and add in chocolate chips or nibs and blend for 15 seconds until they are smaller pieces. Pour into a cup and enjoy with a reusable straw!

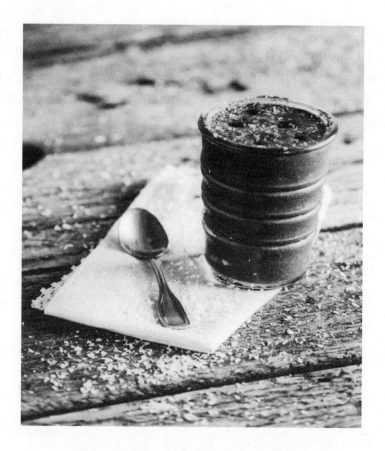

I Heart Blueberries Smoothie

I really do love blueberries. Whether enjoying them fresh or in this delightful smoothie, they are a staple in my life and self-care. You see, blueberries are full of antioxidants and they give me bursts of energy. Try them for yourself and see. I also have a lot of smoothies and I love to have ones that are creamy without the bananas. This has become my favorite creamy banana-less smoothie.

Serves 1 (16 oz.) smoothie
Prep Time: 5 minutes
GF

Ingredients:

- 1 cup blueberries
- 2 coco cubes (coconut milk frozen in ice tray; can omit)
- 1 date
- 1 cup non-dairy milk

In a Vitamix™ or other blender, add all ingredients and blend for about 45 seconds. Enjoy right away. Sometimes I remove half of the milk and blend it. You can use this as the base for a blueberry bowl and top with fresh bananas and granola.

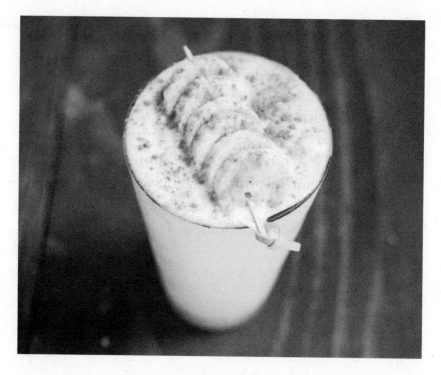

Monkey Milk

Monkey Milk is just bananas and non-dairy milk whipped up in a blender. It's simple, yet so delish. The first time I had it was at a small little raw cafe in California and I was hooked. Seeing that we always have bananas in Hawaii, it's a summer breakfast staple. It also serves as the base for endless smoothie possibilities.

Sometimes I add kale, other times, berries. I have also added cocoa powder to make it chocolatey and no one has ever been mad at me for adding in peanut butter.

Serves 1 (16 oz.) smoothie
Prep Time: 2 minutes
GF

Ingredients:
- 1 cup organic sliced frozen bananas
- 1 cup non-dairy milk

In a Vitamix™ or blender mix bananas with milk starting on slow, gradually taking it to high. Add any other ingredients you want.

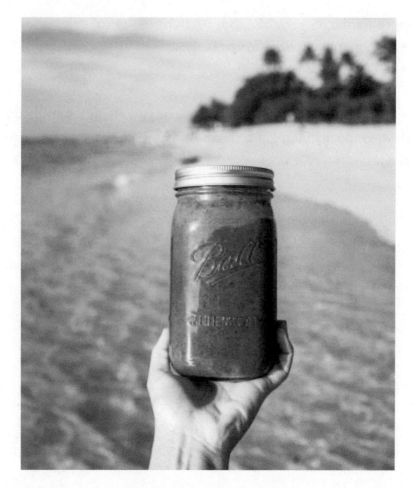

Mixed Berry Smoothie

My body loves berries. They are antioxidant rich, nutrient dense and taste sweet. This is a smoothie I have weekly. This smoothie has everything: fat, fiber, minerals, glucose from fruit, and if you add a scoop of vegan protein powder, you have a tall, dark, and handsome smoothie.

Serves 1 (16 oz.) smoothie
Prep Time: 3 minutes
GF

Ingredients:
- 1 frozen banana (about ½ cup)
- 1 cup frozen mixed berries
- 2 leaves of kale
- 2 tbsp. almond butter
- 1 cup almond milk

In a blender, add milk and all other ingredients, then blend until everything is incorporated. Enjoy and top with a small kale leaf or frozen blueberries. I love to give it a dollop of almond butter on top as well!

TO GO TIP
Pour it in a mason jar with a lid.

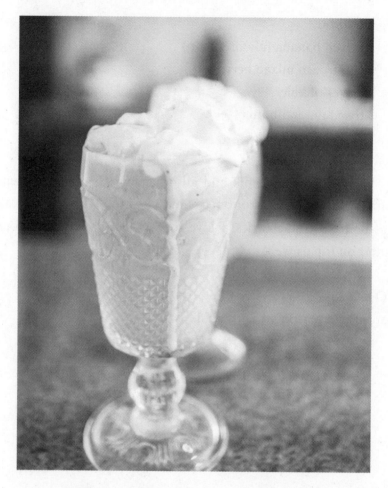

PB and Strawberry Smoothie

I love smoothies, it's like I'm having something naughty, but it's really nice. This smoothie is what I have a few times a week, instead of a sweet treat. It is also perfect for a hot summer day!

Serves 1 (16 oz.) smoothie
Prep Time: 3 minutes
GF

Ingredients:

- 1 cup frozen strawberries
- 2 dates
- 2 tbsp. peanut butter
- 1 cup macadamia nut milk

In a blender, add milk and all other ingredients, then blend until everything is incorporated. For a truly decadent (but healthy!) smoothie, top with coco whipped cream. See recipe below.

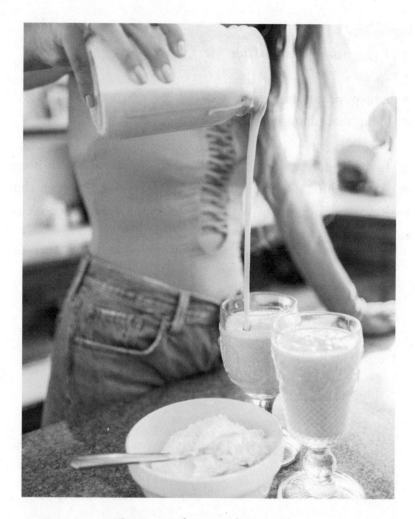

Coco Whipped Cream

Makes 8 servings
Prep Time: 5 minutes
GF

Ingredients:
- 1 can full fat coconut milk (refrigerated)
- 2 tbsp. sugar

In a mixer, scoop out coconut fat and discard water (this will happen naturally if it is cold).

Using a whisk attachment, bring it up to high and beat the coconut fat, adding in the sugar slowly. Once it is whipped into cream, remove and store in the fridge.

PRO TIP

Add chocolate chips and fresh banana slices for an even yummier treat.

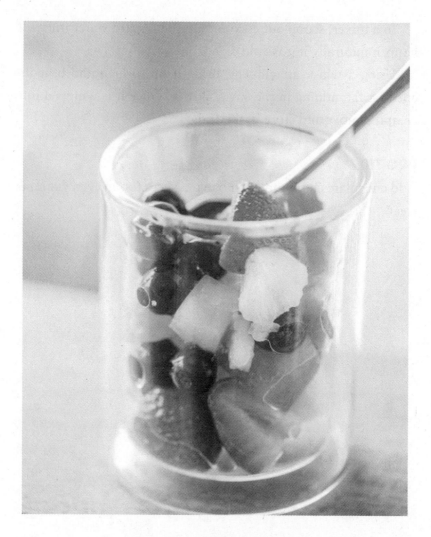

Yummy Yummy Fruit Salad

I love fruit in the morning. I love fruit, period. This is one of my favorite ways to enjoy it outside of a smoothie. Make a bowl and choose to snack on it throughout the day. Add or omit whatever you love or don't. This way you can always guarantee you are getting healthy fruit daily!

Use any fruit that is in season. Cut up enough of the following fruits.

Serves 2
Prep Time: 10 minutes
GF

These are some of my favorites:
- Papaya
- Watermelon
- Strawberries
- Pineapple
- Banana
- Blueberries
- Apple

Cup up fruits into bite-sized pieces, add to a bowl, and serve. You can store it in the fridge for up to 2 days.

Another option: Make it a fruit cocktail by thawing a frozen acai or pitaya pack and pouring it over fruit. This adds beautiful color and extra antioxidants as well.

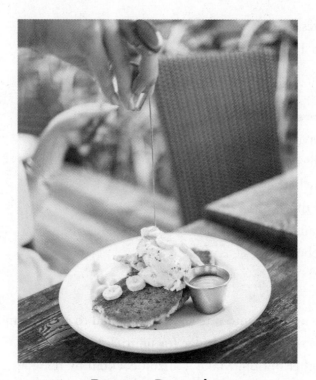

Banana Pancakes

Jack Johnson made banana pancakes famous with his song. I made them vegan. In Hawaii, we have bananas year-round, and I need to find creative ways to use them. I love these because they're gluten free and egg free, but you won't even be able to tell.

Makes 12 Pancakes
Prep Time: 25 minutes
GF

Wet Ingredients:

- 2 cups mashed bananas (the riper the sweeter)
- 1 ½ cups water
- ⅓ cup olive oil
- 1 tbsp. maple syrup

Dry Ingredients:

- 2 cups brown rice flour
- 1 tsp. baking powder
- ½ tsp. baking soda
- 1 ½ tsp. xanthan gum
- ½ tsp. salt

Pour your wet ingredients into the bottom of a bowl or mixer. Add in dry ingredients and stir until everything is incorporated. Warm a sauté pan or griddle on medium heat and add vegan butter or oil. Pour ⅓ cup batter into the pan. Let cook on one side until bubbles form and flip to cook the other side. Repeat until the batter is all gone.

Serve with vegan butter and maple syrup. Fresh fruit and toppings are always welcome.

PRO TIP

Make pancakes and then freeze them in a Ziploc bag so you can put them in your toaster oven to have homemade pancakes without the work and dishes.

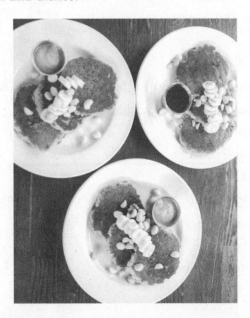

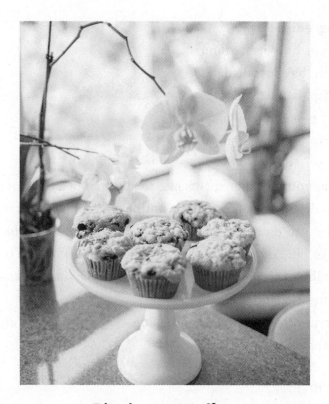

Blueberry Muffins

Makes 12 muffins
Prep Time: 10 minutes

Muffin Ingredients:
- 3 cups flour (all purpose or for gluten-free (brown rice flour or oat flour) and 2 tsp. xanthan gum)
- 1 cup coconut sugar
- 2 tsp. baking powder
- ½ tsp. baking soda
- ½ cup maple syrup
- 2 ½ cups non-dairy milk
- ½ cup olive oil
- 1 ½ cups frozen blueberries

Crumb Topping Ingredients:
- ⅓ cup vegan butter or shortening
- ¼ cup coconut sugar
- 1 tsp. cinnamon
- ⅓ cup flour

Preheat the oven to 375 °F. In a mixer or bowl add all of the ingredients except for the blueberries and mix it until it looks like a thicker pancake batter. Gently add in blueberries to batter. Scoop ½ cup batter into a 12-piece regular-sized muffin pan.

Using a separate clean bowl, mix together crumb topping ingredients and sprinkle on top of muffins before putting into the oven. Bake for 15–18 minutes at 375 °F.

PRO TIP
Use a toothpick to determine if your muffins are baked through. Put the toothpick into the muffin, and if it comes out clean, you are good to go!

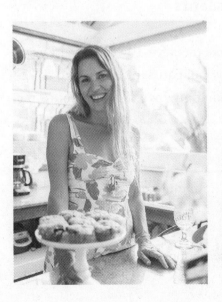
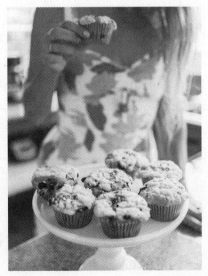

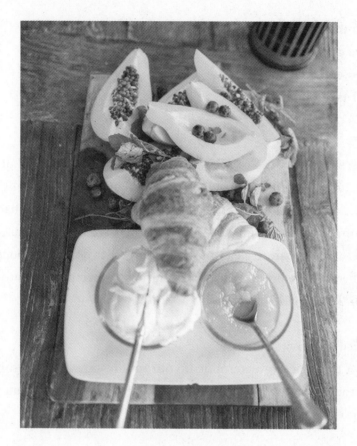

Croissants

I love croissants, and I didn't have them for 10 years after I went vegan. Once in Paris, I found a vegan patisserie and tasted a vegan croissant, I had to start making my own. Say oui-oui to the foods you love healthier!

Makes 12
Prep Time: 1 day ahead and 45 minutes day of

Ingredients:
- 2 (0.25 oz.) packets or 4 ½ teaspoons active dry yeast
- 1 cup lukewarm water

- 3 ½ cups bread flour
- ¼ cup sugar
- 2 tsp. salt (reduce to 1 tsp. if your butter is salted)
- 6 tbsp. vegan butter, softened
- 1 cup vegan butter, softened

Day One

In the bowl of a kitchen stand mixer, add yeast, warm water, and sugar. Let it sit for 10 minutes, until foamy. Meanwhile, combine the dry ingredients. Add dry ingredients plus 6 tablespoons of softened vegan butter to yeast and mix with paddle attachment until dough forms a ball. Switch to dough hook attachment and knead dough for 6–10 minutes. It should be bouncy. Cover and allow to rise in a warm place for 1–2 hours. Dough should be somewhere between double and triple in size.

After it has risen, punch it down and fold into a rectangular shape. Wrap the dough in plastic, or place in a sealed container and refrigerate overnight. Shape 1 cup of softened butter into a square about 6" × 6", using either a sheet of parchment or a small sandwich bag. Refrigerate overnight.

Day Two

The following day, roll dough out into a large rectangle roughly 8" × 16". (Exact measurements aren't important; it just needs to be slightly larger than twice the length of the butter slab.) Place the butter slab on one side and fold dough over to envelop the butter. Pinch around the edges to seal in the butter tightly.

Roll dough out to roughly 24" × 9" (again, this measurement is just a guideline) and perform a double turn: Fold both ends of the dough into the center, and fold in half again to create 4 layers. Roll dough out again to 24" × 9" and perform another double turn. Cover dough and refrigerate for 1 hour.

Cut the dough in two and work with half at a time, leaving the rest in the refrigerator. Roll out to roughly 18" × 9" and use a sharp knife to cut into triangles (for classic croissants). Cut each sheet of dough into thirds (6" × 9" rectangles). Then, cut each rectangle diagonally, corner-to-corner, to create 6 triangles.

Cut a small slit at the base of each triangle and roll your croissant, pushing outward gently with your palms while rolling to elongate the croissant.

Place on a lined baking tray with the point or seam of the croissant on the bottom. Optionally, brush your croissants with 1 tablespoon agave or maple syrup mixed with 2 tablespoons of plant milk to achieve a glossy finish. (Keep the extra; you will brush them one more time.)

Allow croissants to rise at room temperature for 1–2 hours, until at least doubled in size.

Bake croissants for 10 minutes at 400 °F, then lower the temperature to 350 °F and bake for another 12–15 minutes. Enjoy them fresh from the oven with vegan butter and jam. Make a vegan sandwich with them. They are also delicious as is.

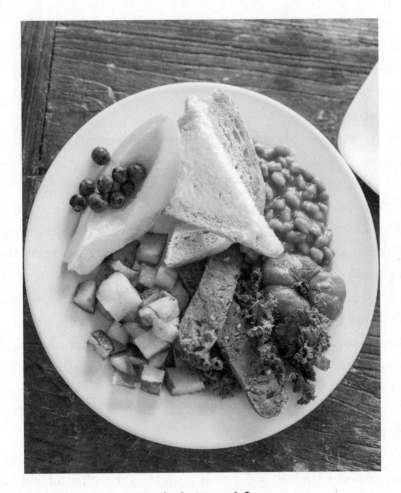

English Breakfast

This is a feast for sharing with friends or family on a lovely summer morning.

The menu includes store bought vegan items, which can be found in almost any grocery store. Pick and choose what you would like to serve. These are quick recipes for a delicious and healthy summer brunch.

Serves 4–8
Prep Time: 45 minutes

Vegan Sausages

Buy 4 vegan sausages. Slice them long ways and bake at 350 °F for ten minutes, or until golden brown.

Toast

Toast 8 slices. My favorite is sourdough topped with vegan butter.

Baked Beans

Buy 2 cans of baked beans. Make sure they are vegan, many baked beans use bacon, but they do indicate if they are vegetarian or vegan friendly.

Roasted Potatoes

Buy 4 russet potatoes. Cut potatoes into half inch cubes and roast with 1 ½ tbsp. olive oil and 2 tsp. salt for 25–30 minutes at 450 °F.

Sautéed Kale

In a sauté pan on medium heat add kale and then add 3 tbsp. water and 1 tsp. salt and give it a stir. Cover with a lid and let water steam it for about 4 minutes. Take off heat and uncover. Serve on a platter.

Baked Tomatoes

Buy 4 tomatoes. Slice them in half along their equator. Lightly sprinkle with salt and pepper. Place tomatoes seed side up on a sheet pan. Bake at 450 °F for 10 minutes. Once they are baked you can top them with fresh herbs if you have them.

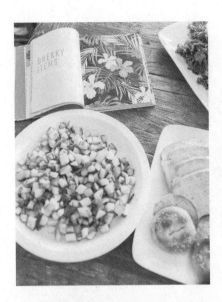

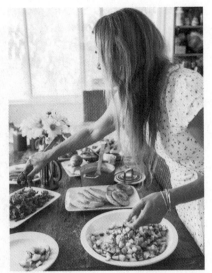

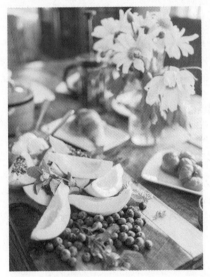

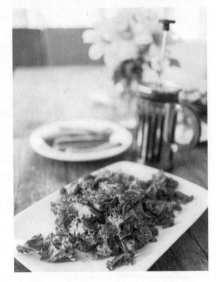

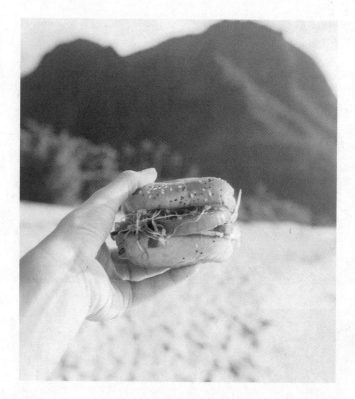

Bagel Sandwich

I love bagels. They are so yummy and toasty. I first had this sandwich in Maui and it quickly became a thing at my house. It is great for breakfast, lunch, or dinner. Serve it up with lots of veggies.

Serves 2
Prep Time: 10 minutes

Ingredients:
- 2 bagels, sliced and toasted
- 2 tbsp. vegan cream cheese
- 2 tbsp. hummus
- ½ cucumber sliced

- 1 tomato sliced
- 2 slices of red onion
- ¼ cup clover sprouts

On your bagel, spread one tablespoon cream cheese and one tablespoon hummus on either bagel slice. Top with onions, cucumbers, tomatoes, and sprouts. Sandwich together. Repeat on the other bagel half.

TO GO TIP

Pack it in a small covered bowl. The bagel fits perfectly inside.

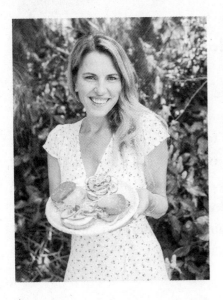
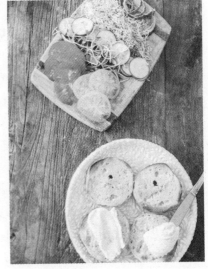

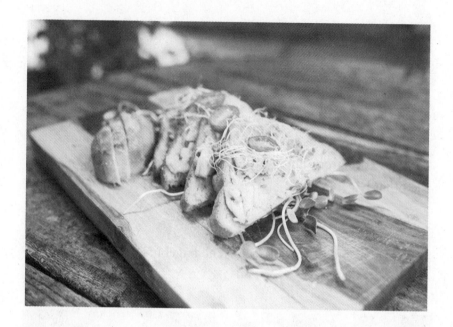

Avocado Toast

It seems like everyone is obsessed with avocado toast these days. You can have it from Hawaii to NY, and it's not just on vegan menus. At the restaurant, we try to have everything be as local as possible, so since avocados are available year-round in Hawaii, putting this on the menu was a no-brainer. Also, can we talk health benefits? They are packed with monounsaturated fatty acids. Avocados are a naturally nutrient-dense food and contain nearly 20 vitamins and minerals.

Serves 2
Prep Time: 10 minutes

Ingredients:
- 4 slices of your favorite bread (gluten-free or not)
- 2 tbsp. vegan butter
- 1 large or 2 small avocados, sliced

- Salt and pepper to taste
- 8 cherry tomatoes (sliced in half)
- ½ cup clover sprouts

Toast your favorite bread and spread butter on it. Next add ¼ of a large avocado or ½ of a small one on each slice of toast. Smoosh avocado on bread. Cut in half on a diagonal and sprinkle with salt and pepper. Top with clover sprouts and tomato garnish.

This recipe is so versatile. Love pickily foods? Top it with pickled radishes and micro greens! Do something fun.

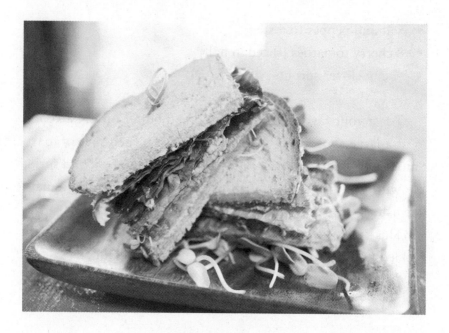

BLT Please

I eat this a lot more than I ever did the original sandwich. I love how savory this brand of "bacon" is. Absolutely delicious, without the bacon.

Serves 1
Prep Time: 15 minutes

Ingredients:
- 2 slices of bread toasted
- ¼ pack of vegan bacon
- 1 or 2 tomatoes slices
- 1 leaf lettuce
- Clover sprouts
- Vegan mayo
- Mustard (optional)

Take vegan bacon out of the package and sauté on each side for about three minutes depending on if you want crispy. Set aside.

Start to construct sandwich bread, vegan mayo (and mustard) on both slices, tomato, lettuce, sprouts, and then bacon.

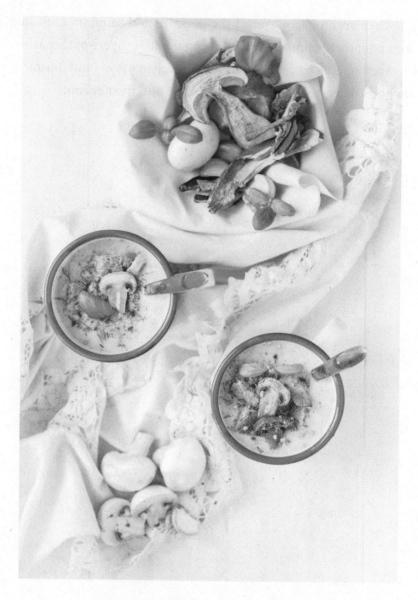

Cream of Mushroom Soup

I could literally eat this soup all day. It is so tasty that even people who don't like mushrooms like it. We use a cashew cream base, which rivals all real cream counterparts. It has a light texture but is super filling. You can substitute any mushrooms.

Serves 6

Prep Time: 25 mins

Ingredients:

- ½ cup onion chopped
- 24 oz. mushrooms quartered
- 3 cups water
- 1 cup cashews
- 2 tsp. salt
- 1 tsp. olive oil

Add olive oil to soup pan on low medium heat and throw in onions. Cook until onions are translucent. Add in mushrooms, water, cashews, and salt. Cook for 15 minutes on low until mushrooms are soft. Take off heat and place in a blender, blend until smooth. Serve warm and enjoy. Keep leftovers in the fridge.

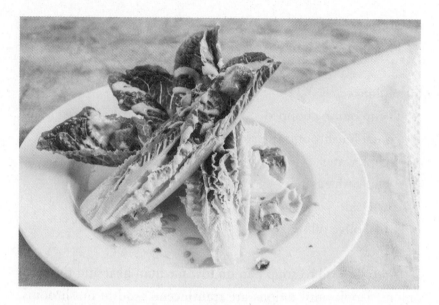

Caesar Salad

I don't know if I ever had a Caesar salad before I was vegan, my friends all love it, but I was freaked out by anchovies. I do, however, remember my first vegan Caesar salad at Cafe Gratitude and it was life changing. Light but filling, crunchy and bready, with a creamy dressing and a hint of lemon.

Serves 4

Prep Time: 15 minutes

Salad Ingredients:
- 2 large or 4 small romaine lettuce heads
- 2 tbsp. nutritional yeast
- A dash of black pepper
- 1 tbsp. capers
- 6 slices gluten-free bread
- 3 tsp. olive oil
- ½ tsp. salt

Dressing Ingredients:

- ½ cup cashews
- ½ cup water
- 2 tbsp. capers
- 1 tbsp. Dijon mustard
- 1 tsp. salt
- Juice of one lemon

Cut bread into ¼ inch squares. Coat in olive oil and salt—bake at 400 °F for 13 minutes or until golden brown. Let cool.

In a blender, mix all dressing ingredients and blend until incorporated. Set aside.

Chop romaine and place in a bowl or platter, sprinkle nutritional yeast and capers, then top with dressing and croutons.

TO GO TIP

Add dressing to the bottom of mason jar, stuff with romaine, capers, nutritional yeast, and top with croutons.

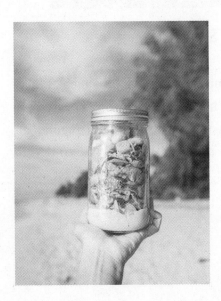
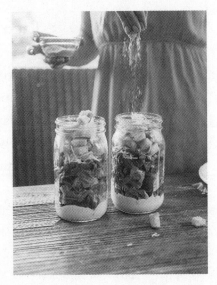

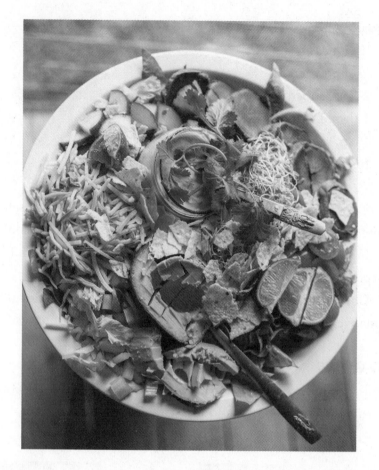

Taco Salad

I love any salads that are able to mask themselves as a meal. I love when they are hearty enough to be a complete meal. This has so many yummy toppings and flavor. It will become a regular at your house. The salad has a few different components, so if you want to get the salad made quickly on the day of, roast your sweet potatoes beforehand.

Serves 4
Prep Time: 20 minutes
GF

Salad Ingredients:
- 2 purple Okinawan sweet potatoes or yams
- ½ pound mixed greens
- 2 grated carrots
- 1 container (8 oz.) cherry tomatoes, halved
- 1 cucumber sliced
- 1 avocado, cubed
- 2 stalks of celery, chopped
- 1 cup crushed tortilla chips
- 2 oz. clover sprouts
- 2 tsp. olive oil
- 1 tsp. salt

Dressing Ingredients:
- ½ cup vegan mayo
- 1 tbsp. ketchup
- 2 tsp. relish

For potatoes or yams. Cube them into 1-inch pieces, toss in olive oil, and salt. Roast at 425 °F for 20 minutes. Set aside.

Wash and prepare all vegetables. Place mixed greens in a large bowl, top with grated carrots, chopped celery, sliced cucumber, sweet potatoes, and halved tomatoes. Combine all dressing ingredients in a cup and stir. Pour onto salad and toss. Top salad with crushed tortilla chips and a handful of sprouts.

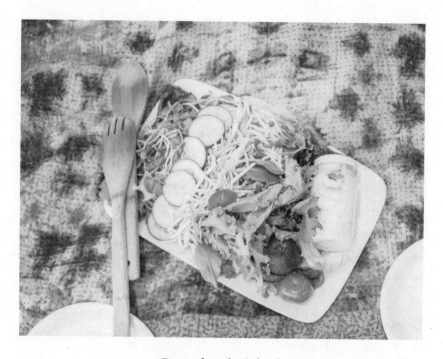

Ranched Salad

I love ranch dressing. In high school, one of my favorite meals was French bread dipped in ranch dressing. So when I learned how to make it vegan, it became a main food group in my life. The healthiest way I have it is with a simple salad. Enjoy.

Serves 4
Prep Time: 10 minutes
GF

Salad Ingredients:
- ½ pound mixed greens
- 2 grated carrots
- 1 large tomato, diced
- 1 cucumber sliced
- 2 oz. sunflower sprouts

Dilly Ranch Dressing Ingredients:
- ½ cup veganaise
- 2 tbsp. water
- 1 tbsp. dill
- 1 tsp. salt

Wash and prepare all vegetables. Place mixed greens in a large bowl, top with grated carrots, sliced cucumber, and diced tomatoes. Combine all dressing ingredients in a cup and stir. Pour onto salad and toss. Top salad with sunflower sprouts, and a little extra dressing, you won't regret it!

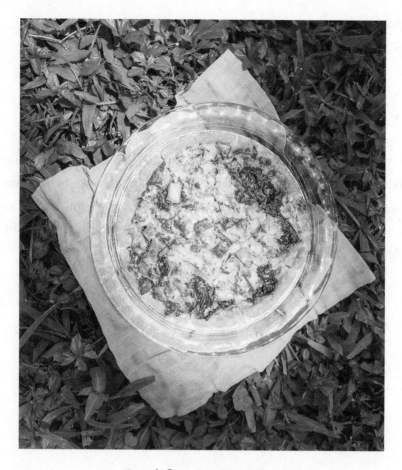

Cauliflower Quiche

This recipe is good for breakfast, lunch, brunch, dinner, or even as a snack. Although it takes a little bit of prep time, it is so worth it. Save some time by buying a premade vegan pie crust at the store, but if you want to impress, make my homemade crust using the recipe below!

Serves 8
Prep Time: 1 hour
No Fail Pie Crust
Makes 2 crusts

Dough Ingredients:

- 2 ½ cups all-purpose flour
- 1 tbsp. sugar
- ½ tsp. salt
- ½ cup vegan butter, cold and cut into pieces
- 2–3 tbsp. ice water

In a mixer or bowl, add in flour, sugar, and salt and mix together. Add in butter and keep mixing until crumbly. Add in ice water slowly and stop mixing as it forms into a dough. If it isn't a dough add in more ice water. YOU DO NOT WANT TO OVER MIX. Use your hands to form dough into two discs. Wrap the dough in parchment or plastic wrap and put in the fridge and let rest for at least 30 minutes.

On a floured surface roll out your dough into a circle with a rolling pin. You can check if it's big enough by holding a pie plate upside down over it. Your dough circle should be as large as the largest circumference of the pie plate. I take my dough circle and fold it into quarters for easy transferring into the pie plate.

Keep in the fridge until ready to bake.

Quiche Filling:

- 1 head cauliflower, chopped into 1-inch pieces
- 2 russet potatoes, chopped into 1-inch pieces
- 2 tbsp. olive oil
- 1 ½ tsp. salt
- ½ cup cashews
- ⅓ cup water
- 2 cups washed spinach

This is a 4-part recipe that can all be done at the same time or prepared the day before and baked the following day.

Cauliflower and spinach

Preheat the oven to 400 °F.

On a sheet pan, lined with parchment, add cauliflower, 1 tbsp. olive oil, and ½ tsp. of salt. Bake for 25 minutes or until golden brown. Remove from the oven and add in spinach. Stir and set aside.

Potatoes

Bring a large pot of water to a boil, add the potatoes and a tsp. of salt. Boil for about 13 minutes or until cooked through. Drain and set aside.

Cashew cheese

In a blender add cashews, water, and the remaining salt. Blend until consistently smooth and creamy.

Final step

In a bowl, mix potatoes, cauliflower and spinach, and the cashew cheese. Scoop half of the mixture into one of the pie crusts. Repeat this step with the other pie crust. Bake at 375 °F for 25 minutes until golden brown on top.

PRO TIP

Cover and freeze one of the quiches for later.

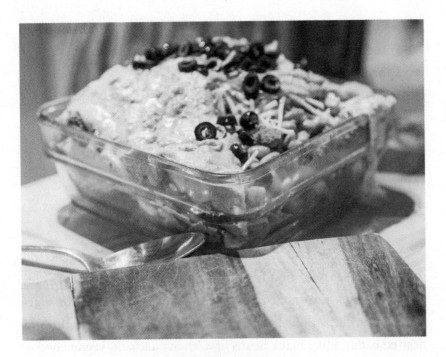

Jackfruit Nachos

Who doesn't crave nachos? Crispy, crunchy, salty, and creamy. Just because you are trying to eat healthier doesn't mean you don't get to enjoy your nachos. Play around with toppings you love. Hot sauce optional.

Serves 6
Prep Time: 25 minutes
GF

Ingredients:
- 5 cups of restaurant style tortilla chips
- ¾ cup vegan cheese
- ¾ cup cooked black beans
- 1 cup shredded jackfruit
- 1 can sliced olives

- ¾ cup tomatoes
- ½ red onion sliced
- 2 tbsp. fresh cilantro chopped
- 1 pack of enchilada or taco seasoning
- ¾ cup cashews
- ½ cup water
- 1 tsp. salt

Preheat oven to 400 °F.

Heat up your black beans in a small saucepan and season with a little sea salt. In a blender, combine cashews, water, salt, and enchilada seasoning pack until creamy, set aside. Next arrange your chips on a large serving platter and add toppings in desired order. I like black beans first, then jackfruit, vegan cheese, tomatoes, olives, and red onion. Bake for 15 minutes. Remove from the oven and top with enchilada cashew cheese and cilantro. Enjoy immediately.

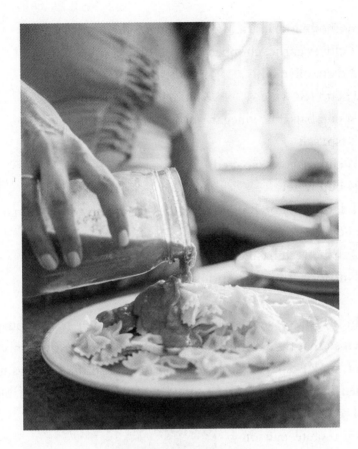

Pasta Marinara

I went to Italy in 2018 and fell in love with pasta all over again. Here's the crazy part—after thinking for years that pasta was making me put on weight, I was in fact losing it. Since I came home, I have eaten a lot of pasta. I just make sure it is organic Italian pasta. The real deal. And making my own sauce is so easy, which I always do now.

Serves 4
Prep Time: 25 minutes
1 bag pasta of choice, cooked in salted, boiling water to perfection

Homemade Marinara Ingredients:

- 2 cloves garlic, chopped
- 2 tbsp. olive oil
- ½ cup red wine
- ¼ cup balsamic vinegar
- 2 tsp. salt
- ⅓ cup cashews (soaked)
- ¼ cup water
- 1 large can of Italian tomatoes or 2 cups fresh tomatoes, chopped
- 2 tbsp. fresh basil chiffonade
- Nutritional yeast to sprinkle on top

In a blender, add cashews (soaked in water for 2 hours to soften so that they blend properly, unless you have a Vitamix™), water, and 1 tsp. salt and blend on high until the cashews have turned into a cream. Add canned or fresh tomatoes and blend until pureed. Set aside.

In a sauté pan on medium heat, add olive oil and garlic and cook for 2 minutes. Add wine and simmer for 2 more minutes. Add tomato, cashew mixture, balsamic, and salt. Cook for about 10 minutes on medium to low heat and then add basil. Serve over pasta and sprinkle with nutritional yeast.

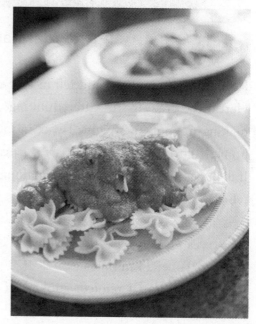

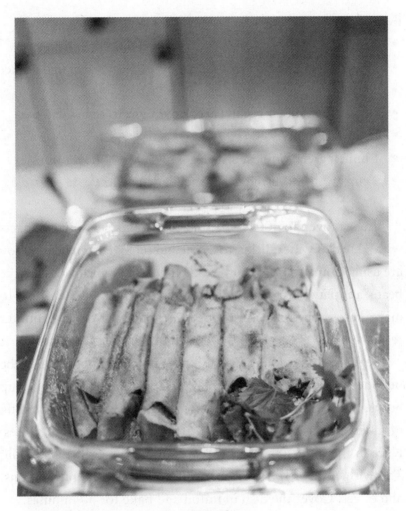

Enchiladas

I love enchiladas so much. They are so yummy, seem fancier than a taco or burrito, and can be made ahead of time. You can make them completely from scratch or use this shortcut recipe and make it easy.

Serves 6
Prep Time: 45 minutes

Ingredients:

- 8 tortillas
- 2 packs of enchilada seasoning (dry) or 2 cans enchilada sauce
- 2 cans beans or 2 cups homemade beans
- 1 bag of shredded vegan cheese
- 1 can black olives, sliced
- 1 bunch green onions, sliced
- 3 cups water (if using dried enchilada packet)

Preheat oven to 400 °F. In a saucepan, mix seasoning packets with 3 cups of water. Bring to a boil and remove from heat. If you are using canned sauce, just heat them up. In a saucepan, heat the beans and have other ingredients prepped to assemble. I like to make sure everything is chopped and lined up on my counter ready to go.

Begin by lining a 9" x 13" dish with parchment paper. Dip the outside of the tortilla in enchilada sauce, and fill with ¼ cup beans, 2 tbsp. vegan cheese, a spoonful of olives, and a sprinkling of green onions. Gently roll the tortilla and tuck in the sides. Place in the dish. Repeat this step until the casserole dish is full. Top with extra enchilada sauce, remaining cheese, green onions, and olives. Cover the dish in tinfoil and bake for 30 minutes.

Cashew Cheese

I love this recipe and I use it as cheese in so many recipes. You could add anything you want to it to make it more creamy. It is the base in our mac n cheese please. If you add sweetener it will act as a baked custard filling. It is in my lasagna, enchilada casserole and any creamy dressing I make that I don't use veganaise for.

Makes 2 ½ cups
Prep Time: 5 minutes

- 2 cups unsalted cashews
- 1 ½ cups water
- 3 tbsp. salt (sub sugar or syrup for sweetness)

Add all of your ingredients in Vitamix™ (or blender) and start to blend on low. Gradually bring up speed to high. Blend until smooth.

You don't need a high-powered blender for this. Just soak your nuts to get them soft first, or speed up this process by boiling your nuts first.

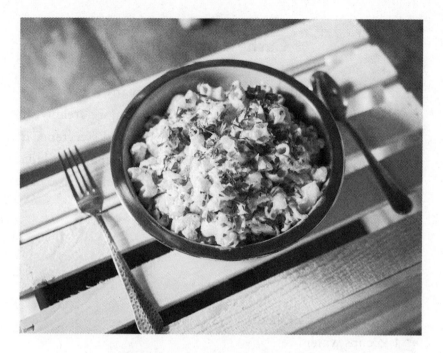

Mac and Cheese Please

Yes please to mac and cheese, but without the dairy and gluten, double please! Have fun and add yummy sautéed vegetables or top with bread crumbs. We use carrots with cashew cheese to create our sauce.

Serves 6
Prep Time: 30 minutes
GF

- 1 package brown rice elbow macaroni
- 1 carrot, cut into thin circles
- 2 cups cashew cheese (see recipe)
- 1 tsp. salt
- Pepper to taste
- Hot sauce optional

Make pasta according to box instructions. Make cashew cheese. In a small pot, boil or steam your carrots until they are soft (for about 10 minutes). Remove from heat and drain. In a blender add carrots to cashew cheese and blend. Once you strain pasta, add it back to the pot and add cashew–carrot cheese. Stir in salt and pepper. Serve hot.

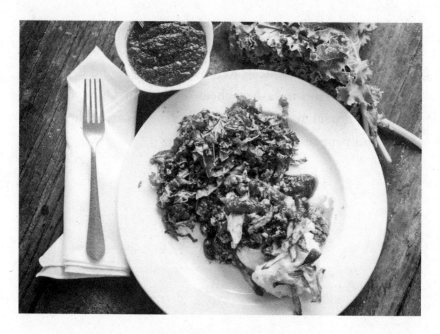

BBQ Cauli-Power

BBQ cauliflower is one of my (and my family's) favorite recipes. I serve with rice or mashed potatoes and sautéed greens for the perfect balance of color and flavor on the plate. Keep leftovers in the fridge to enjoy as a snack all week. Perfect snack for a ride in the country on the weekend.

Serves 4
Prep Time: 40 minutes
GF

Ingredients:
- 1 head cauliflower (large) chopped into one inch pieces
- ¼ red onion chopped
- 4 tbsp. olive oil
- 1 tbsp. salt
- 3 tbsp. dill

BBQ Sauce Ingredients:

- 1 cup ketchup
- 2 tbsp. maple syrup
- 1 tsp. vinegar (rice or apple cider)
- 1 tsp. dark chili powder
- 2 tbsp. olive oil
- 3 tbsp. water
- Dash of salt

For BBQ sauce, place all ingredients in a blender and gradually bring it up to high until all ingredients are blended together. Use right away or store in a mason jar for up to two months in the fridge.

Preheat the oven to 400 °F.

Chop cauliflower into one-inch pieces. Chop ¼ onion.

Mix all the ingredients (except BBQ sauce) together in a bowl and put into a 9" x 13" baking dish. Roast in an oven for 30 minutes, then remove and coat in BBQ sauce.

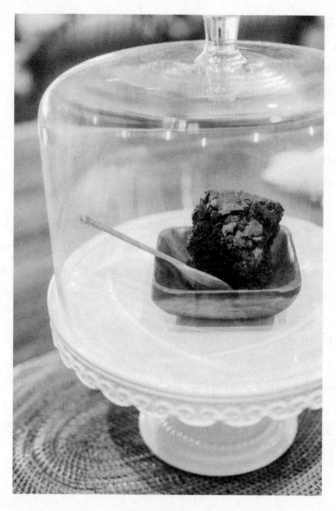

Brownies

Free of gluten, wheat, soy, dairy, and eggs but full of flavor and love! Don't ask why, just try and you will never doubt me again. This is indulgence at its finest!

Makes 12
Prep Time: 45 minutes
GF

Ingredients:

- 2 cups brown rice flour
- 2 cups sugar
- 1 cup cocoa powder
- 2 tsp. baking powder
- 1 ½ tsp. xanthan gum
- 1 tsp. baking soda
- 1 tsp. salt
- ½ cup oil
- 1 ½ cup water

Preheat oven to 350 °F. Mix the dry ingredients together using a stand mixer or whisk, and then slowly add in water and oil and mix until just blended. Pour the mixture into a 9" × 13" pan lined with parchment paper. Smooth with a spatula and top with chocolate chips. Bake for 40 minutes and voila! You have made delicious vegan brownies. Let cool before cutting.

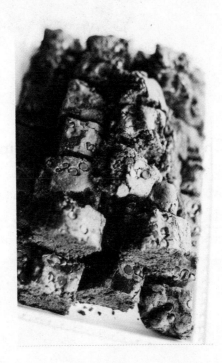

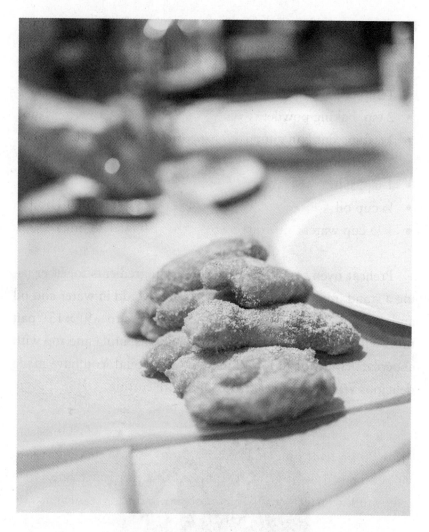

Churros with Chocolate Dip

Who doesn't love a fair? I always think of all the yummy greasy fried sweet foods. Now you can enjoy one of my favorites, churros, without getting a tummy ache after. They are easily made gluten-free.

Serves 4–6
Prep Time: 15 minutes

Dough Ingredients:

- 1 ¼ cup oil (vegetable or canola oil)
- 1 cup + 3 tbsp. sugar (reserve 3 tbsp. for the end)
- 1 tbsp. cinnamon
- 2 cups water
- 2 cups all-purpose flour (gluten-free if needed)

Chocolate Dip Ingredients:

- ½ cup cocoa powder
- 1 ½–2 tbsp. maple syrup

Bring 2 cups of water and ¼ cup oil to a boil in a saucepan. Add 3 tbsp. sugar and the 2 cups of flour. Stir until the mixture becomes a ball of dough. Remove dough and add to mixer and beat for ½ minutes to add air in. You could also use an electric hand mixer for this step. Transfer the dough to a pastry bag with a large star tip. Pipe out 4-inch churros.

On medium heat, bring remaining oil to a low boiling point. Add in dough, flipping after 1 minute on each side. Remove and place on paper towels to soak up some of the oil.

Mix remaining sugar and cinnamon in a bowl. Dip the fried churros in the mixture and plate to serve.

To make the chocolate dip simply mix the cocoa powder and maple syrup with a fork until combined.

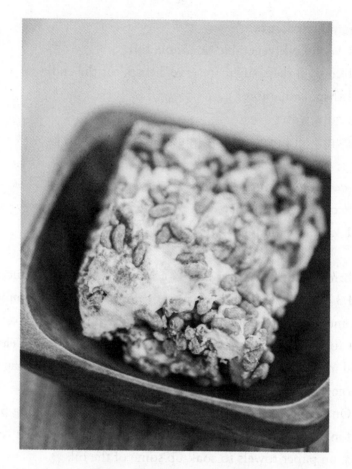

Riced Crispy Treats

Is it even possible to not love riced crispy treats? They are light, crispy, and always a crowd pleaser. This recipe requires no baking, so it makes them easy to make on the fly. There are so many different vegan marshmallows and organic rice cereals these days. It really is easier than ever to make vegan riced crispy treats.

Makes 12 giant treats
Prep Time: 15 minutes
GF

- 1 box organic rice cereal (8 ½ cups)
- 2 packages (10 oz.) vegan marshmallows
- 4 tbsp. vegan butter
- 9" x 13" pan, covered in parchment paper.

Plastic wrap or gloves to press the final product down

Melt butter in a large steel stockpot on medium.

Turn down to medium–low heat, add vegan marshmallows and stir. Keep heat low so that marshmallows melt rather than burn.

Once almost all the marshmallows are melted, add in rice cereal. Continue stirring.

Transfer to the parchment lined pan and use plastic wrap or gloves to press the treats down with your hands. You want to make the treats condensed and solid so they stay together. Let the treat cool down. Cut into 12 squares and serve! Keep covered on the counter.

Chapter 7

SUPERFOODS = SUPERPOWERS

An Introduction to Some of the Most Powerful Foods in the World

As I have discussed throughout this book, the food you eat creates your mood and sets the baseline for your overall health. Eating healthy foods will jump start your cells and boost your energy because the cells in your body convert food into nutrients and nutrients into energy. When you eat a standard American diet, your intake of processed foods, high-fat dairy products, refined grains, corn, high-fructose corn syrup, fried foods, and butter supports disease and takes away your vitality.

Remember, we are what we eat.

One of the reasons I have been able to continue with an organic, vegan diet for so long is because I know I can have all the foods I love in a healthier form.

The research shows that incorporating mostly organic, plant-based foods supports our health and immunity. You don't need to be at 100% to improve your life. You're going to find that even a small step is a big win because it will improve the way you feel. Nothing has supported my health more than going vegan. Fifteen years and I still feel like I have control over my health and can build my immunity through my food and life choices, each and every day. You can too! Are you ready to own your health and wellness? Your decision to start is the first step. It's easier and more fun than you've ever imagined. Let's do this!

Let's talk about superfoods. They are super for your health.

Your New Love Playlist

Lemony Garlic Ginger Vinaigrette
Turmeric Shots
Feel the Burn Ginger Shot
Blueberry Overnight Oats
I Love You Matcha Latte
Nutty Almond Mylk
Green Dream Spinach Smoothie
4-Layered Smoothie

Superfoods have superpowers.

Fruits and veggies are like a rainbow of vitamins and minerals that are food for your cells. Healthy cells = healthy immune system. Juices, elixirs, and smoothies can deliver a power punch of concentrated vitamins, minerals, and antioxidants. Start using food as medicine. What can we do to internally boost our immune system to protect ourselves from illness?

Here are 8 super immune-boosting ingredients and a recipe to go with each one.

Food has the ability to turn disease on and off, here are ways to reset and eat healthy.

1. GARLIC

2. TURMERIC

3. GINGER

4. BLUEBERRIES

5. MATCHA

6. ALMONDS

7. SPINACH

8. SPIRULINA

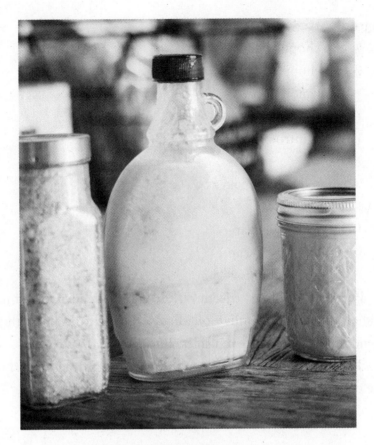

Recipe for Garlic

Raw garlic is magnificent at giving your body's immune system a helping hand. It has natural antibacterial and anti-inflammatory properties, helping you ward off illness. It is so good for overall health.

Lemony Garlic Ginger Vinaigrette
This recipe zings up any salad and adds so much flavor.

Makes: 2 ½ cups dressing
Prep Time: 15 minutes
GF

Ingredients:
- ¼ cup chopped ginger
- ⅓ cup chopped garlic
- ⅓ cup lemon juice
- 1 tsp. dijon mustard
- 1 tsp. cilantro
- 1 tsp. salt
- ¼ tsp. red pepper flakes
- 1 cup olive oil
- 1 cup of rice vinegar
- ⅓ cup of maple syrup

Put all ingredients, except olive oil, in a blender. Blend until mixed and then add olive oil slowly through the lid with the blender on low until it emulsifies. Enjoy it on any salad.

This lasts in the fridge for up to 3 months. Just let it warm on the counter if olive oil gets cold and solidifies at all.

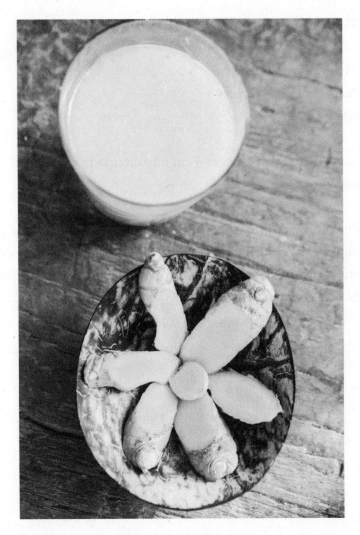

Turmeric Shots

Turmeric is amazing. It is anti-viral, anti-bacterial, anti-inflam-
mation, good for your heart, and that's the very short list of its
magic traits. Turmeric grows abundantly in Hawaii, so I always
have it at my fingertips. If you don't live in Hawaii or by a Whole
Foods™, you can use the powder form instead. But remember,
fresh is always best. You will need a juicer for this recipe. But you
can always blend with a little water and then strain.

Turmeric Shots

Makes two 2-oz. shots
Prep Time: 10 minutes
GF

* ¼ cup turmeric peeled and cut into chunks that will fit in your juicer.

Put pieces into your juicer and make according to your juicer's directions. Take as a shot, I do 2 oz. at a time. You can dilute it with water or lemon juice. Turmeric is the superstar of superfoods. Cheers to your health.

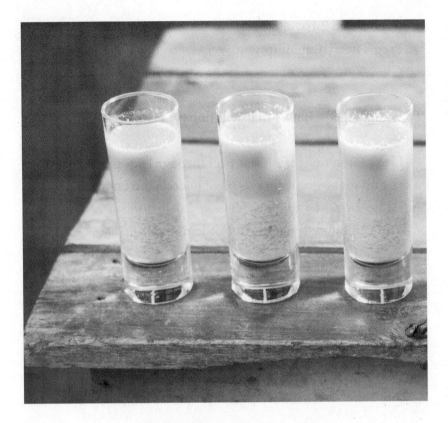

Feel the Burn Ginger Shot

The spicy, aromatic ginger root is used to add some kick to drinks, teas, soups, and Asian dishes, and it's also a real super-food. Ginger reduces inflammation and supports your immune system.

Feel the Burn Ginger Shots

I love ginger. It has so many health benefits and I always feel better when I drink it. At some point, I stopped taking shots at the bar and replaced them with health shots. You can always dilute it if you prefer it to be not as strong as I like them. I like to feel it burn and work its magic. You will need a juicer for this recipe or you can always use a blender with a little water and then strain.

Makes two 2-oz. shots
Prep Time: 10 minutes
GF

- ¼ lb. ginger (chunks that will fit in your juicer)

I leave skin on if fresh but peel if rough. Put pieces into your juicer and make according to your juicer's directions. Take as a shot, I do 2 oz. at a time.

You can dilute it with water or lemon juice.

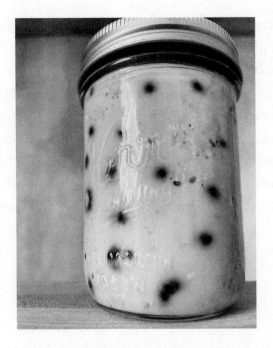

Blueberries

These little purple balls are full of antioxidants and phytoflavinoids. Blueberries are also high in potassium and vitamin C. They have been shown to lower your risk of heart disease. As if that wasn't enough, they are also anti-inflammatory.

Blueberry Overnight Oats

Serves 1
Prep Time: 5 minutes
GF

- 1 cup almond milk
- 1 cup rolled oats
- ¼ cup fresh or frozen blueberries
- 1–2 tsp. maple syrup (depending on how sweet you like it)

This recipe is so easy and quick, it literally takes two minutes to throw it all together!

In a mason jar, mix together all the ingredients.

Close the lid, shake the jar, and refrigerate overnight or for at least 4–5 hours.

You can always use a bowl and spoon for mixing as well. I love the mason jar because they are "to go" or "for here."

In the morning, stir the oats and add a splash of milk for a thinner consistency, then top with fresh blueberries and cinnamon.

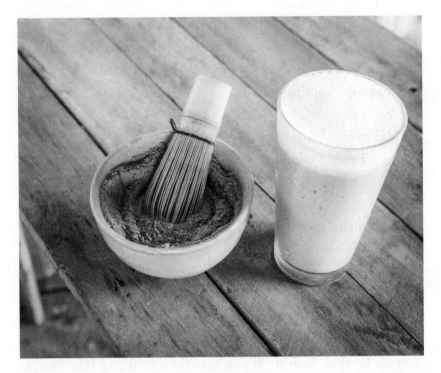

Matcha

Matcha green tea powder boosts the immune system due to its high antioxidant content. Particularly, epigallocatechin gallate (EGCG) assists your body's production of T-cells, which reduce inflammation and fight pathogens.

I Love You Matcha Latte

Matcha is amazing! It is green tea but is thicker like coffee. It packs a punch of flavor that will remind you of green tea ice cream from your favorite Japanese restaurant. It is full of antioxidants and all studies point to a long list of benefits. In just one bowl of Matcha there are substantial quantities of potassium, vitamins A and C, iron, protein, and calcium. I love when something that tastes so yummy supports your body and cells. When you mix it into a latte with hemp milk you are getting a power punch of protein.

Matcha is also a great replacement when you are trying to give up coffee, and, just like coffee, there are so many varieties of matcha that you need to try different brands until you find the one that suits your taste buds.

Makes one 16-oz. latte
Prep Time: 7 minutes
GF

- 2 tsp. matcha powder
- ¼ cup hot water
- 2 tsp. organic sugar or maple syrup
- 12 oz. hemp milk

As you see in the picture, we have some special tools, a Japanese tea bowl and whisk. If you have these tools, add the matcha and sugar to the bowl and add hot water and whisk for 45 seconds. Heat milk in a pan on medium heat and use whisk to create a little foam. Heat until you reach the desired temp. Pour hot milk into a mug, stir in matcha mixture. If you don't have a bowl and whisk, use a cereal bowl and fork. Adjust the sugar amount to your liking. During summer/warm months don't heat milk, and fill your mug with ice, pour in the milk and then the matcha. Enjoy!

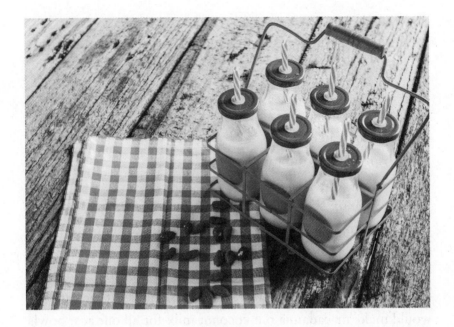

Almonds

Almonds are high in vitamin E, which acts as an antioxidant in your body and helps the immune system to function.

Nutty Almond Mylk

It is so simple to make your own milk. You literally blend water with nuts or seeds and strain. I like adding in a little maple syrup for sweetness.

I use almond milk as my main milk. So anything you use milk in, I use almond milk in. I find it versatile and my body loves it and my recipes come out great. Almonds are naturally alkalizing, so... so is this. You can change the recipe to suit your taste buds; more almonds, more water, but this is how I like it.

I use a nut milk bag to strain it—you can find these for sale at most health food stores. If you can't, a a paint strainer from a hardware store will work or you can just use a clean dish towel to strain it.

Makes 2 quarts
Prep Time: 5 minutes
GF

- 1 cup of organic raw almonds
- 7 cups of water
- 2 tbsp. maple syrup (optional)

In a Vitamix™ or blender, mix almonds with water, gradually taking it to high. You want to pulverize those almonds. Next, strain through the nut milk bag into a large bowl. Transfer to a pitcher and store in the fridge. Will last 4 days in your fridge.

You can replace any nut or seed for almonds. At the cafe, we would make macadamia nut coconut milk for all our acai bowls and smoothies. I have tried and love cashews, sesame seeds, and coconut, and they all are tasty in their own way. Have fun and find the one that makes your taste buds happy.

There are many things you can do with the leftover pulp; however, these days I compost it.

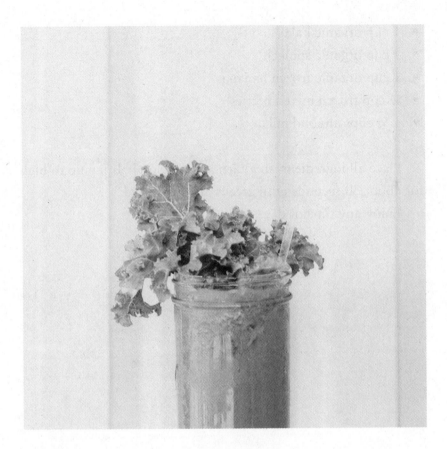

Spinach

Spinach is packed with numerous antioxidants and beta carotene, which may increase the infection-fighting ability of our immune systems.

Green Dream Spinach Smoothie

Love yourself enough to give yourself greens any time of day.
The sweetest way to get your greens.

Makes two 12-oz. smoothies
Prep Time: 6 minutes
GF

- 1 cup organic kale
- 1 cup organic spinach
- 1 cup organic frozen bananas
- ½ cup frozen mixed berries
- 1 ½ cups almond milk

Place all ingredients in a blender and slowly bring up to high for about 30 seconds until greens are pulverized.

Enjoy any time of day.

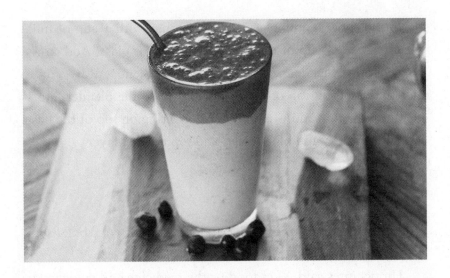

Spirulina

Spirulina contains potent nutrients known as polysaccharides, which are widely regarded to be a powerful immune system booster, assisting in the prevention of a wide variety of maladies.

4-Layered Smoothie

Makes two 12-oz. smoothies
Prep Time: 10 minutes
GF

Ingredients:
- 1 cup frozen bananas
- ½ cup frozen strawberries
- ½ cup frozen pitaya (dragon fruit)
- ½ cup frozen blueberries
- 1 ½ cups almond milk
- 1 tsp. frozen spirulina

In a blender, combine 1 cup of bananas with 1 cup of milk. Blend. Scoop ½ cup of the smoothie into your glass. Add strawberries to the blender with ¼ cup of milk. Blend. Add ⅓ cup to glass, layering on top of base. Add pitaya to the blender and ¼ cup milk. Blend. Add ⅓ cup to glass, layering on top of the base. Add in spirulina and blueberries and top the last layer.

Serve with a straw.

Add these foods to your diet to help support your body's immune response.

Hippocrates said, «Let food be thy medicine and medicine be thy food.»

These SUPERFOODS are preventative medicine. They are called super because of how much nutrition they hold by weight. If you can't get them in a fresh form, get powders and such. Also remember, not too little and not too much. You want to add these antioxidant heroes into your life, but not go overboard.

Now let's talk about where to go from here.

Gentle reminder,
stumble with grace.

Chapter 8

SO WHAT, NOW WHAT?

How to Make it a Lifestyle and Stay in it

L isten, writing this book changed me. There was so much I had forgotten in the last 16 years. I became complacent and stopped showing up for myself in the best way I know how for me. The writing of this book was the reminder I needed. My sister Aisha, who helps me with all my writing, is a teacher and I couldn't have done it without her. She has said that this book has motivated her and opened her eyes. It was a reminder of where we can divorce habits and break up with beliefs that are not serving us. A reminder of where we make excuses or let laziness of mind get us stuck into it being "good enough." I want to remind you, it can get better from where you are. It can be better from where I am. Writing this book became the compass to help us find the road to where we can be healthier human beings. All I can hope is that it has changed you. Considering I have been on this journey for quite some time, let me be the example of "never thinking you know and becoming complacent". Read up on what areas of health you are interested in. After writing this book, I am looking at areas of my life that need improvement.

This leads me to feedback. Are you open to giving yourself feedback? I had to be honest with myself when I was writing this book. I am not perfect and there have been times where I fell off the horse in a lot of areas of my health. I need reminders. I need others' experience and expertise to continue growing and nourishing myself, both nutritionally and spiritually.

Let's get real, if we are honest with ourselves, humans love feedback, mostly positive. There is no one that will give you better, more honest feedback than yourself. It's so important to be honest with yourself. In the beginning, you may need to check in regularly to see if you showed up and kept the promises to yourself. A lot of times, we are searching for feedback from others, but we are the truest holders of the knowledge we need to feel good.

Nothing makes you look more inward at yourself than a divorce. While friends and accountability can be helpful, they will never know what is truly going on inside YOUR body or mind. Now that your ex, the diets, are out, are you willing to look and see what you want for yourself and whether or not you are setting up those goals and meeting them. It is called self-responsibility. By no means am I saying you need to be perfect, or that you have to do this on your own, but it feels so much better when you know you are doing your best and feeling your best for you.

Daily Inventory

This is a way to take inventory of how you are showing up. RESPONSIBILITY IS KEY. You must learn your blind spots. You will be able to track how you are doing in whatever areas you want to shift this week. You can choose as few, or as many, as you want.

Start in the a.m., with a list of areas in your life that are important to you.

Example:

I look at things like:

- Diet
- Exercise
- Overall health
- Self-care
- Mental health
- Doing the work
- Relationships

Tonight, make a list of the areas and score yourself 1–5 (1 = nothing and 5 = nailed it)

Add notes on what went right or wrong that day.

Start looking for patterns in your life and notice where you give up or let go, and where you are all in.

You know your habits better than anyone else, and you know who you want to be. Start to connect the dots and make new patterns where necessary.

Being honest and giving feedback to yourself will help you see what you have to bridge in your life to get closer to where you want to be.

Scoring example:

- Diet (4 out of 5)
  - I ate healthy but had some vegan cookies after lunch.

- Exercise (5 out of 5)
  - Pilates and walk!

- Overall health (4 out of 5)
  - I feel great.

- Self-Care (4 out of 5)
  - Did a long face mask and went to the beach.

- Mental Health (3 out of 5)
  - Didn't meditate. Going to tomorrow.

- Doing the work (5 out of 5)
  - I'm here.

- Relationships (3 out of 5)
  - Didn't put much into relationships today, but they are all good.

This helps me stay on my goals in all areas of my life. It helps keep me out of disease.

Dis-ease is such a tricky thing, if you break it down, it means you are not in ease. If you have disease in your body, then your body is not at ease. There are so many issues in the world and different things that cause diseases. The reason I decided to talk about food is because food is what helps create your defenses to all the outside threats (your immune system). If we're talking about self-responsibility, truly feeding our body is a responsibility we have for our health. This is the relationship you have with food and why you want to divorce your diet.

I have found that the only way to know what your body needs is to educate yourself on how your body works, what it needs, and to start replacing your fave foods with ingredients that bring you to life. As I have stated, you do not need to be vegan to be healthy. However, adding more plants to your life is a key to unlocking your health. Here are some ways to help you be more plant-centered.

Have a WHY

Why do you want to eat this way and what is it you want to change? This WHY will become your North Star and compass. Create a list, have something you can go back to when you need motivation.

Educate yourself on the meat and dairy industry

There are so many videos, and books on the meat and dairy industry. Check out my Amazon™ list for books I love. Go to Netflix™ for inspirational and eye-opening films like, *The Game Changers, What the Health, and Forks Over Knives.*

Baby Steps

What is one thing you can change today? Is it ordering almond milk at your local coffee shop? Eliminating some non-vegan items from your fridge? Start small and do a little more every day and week. Take it one step at a time!

Eat until you are full!

You are transitioning into a healthier lifestyle full of more fruits and veggies than ever before. Almost all plant-based foods tend to be lower in calories, so, by weight, you need more food. If you are not full after a meal, you can have some more. Your body is adjusting to a new variety of foods, give it some grace.

Concentrate on nutrient-based whole foods

There are many "accidentally vegan" items, like your favorite sandwich cookies. While it is fun to treat yourself every once in a while, you s should try to get as many nutrient-dense foods into your system as you can. Eat the rainbow! When in doubt, add veggies like kale to your smoothies.

Replace it!

Don't give up everything you love! There are so many vegan replacements for the foods you enjoy. There are vegan mayos, faux meats, crackers, and mac and cheese. Figure out which ones you like and stock up.

When I'm feeling lost or powerless, I have some important food reminders that I always come back to...

- Water yourself
  - Water is one of the most cleansing ingredients we have on the planet. Now that you are eating a more fibrous, nutrient-dense diet, you will need to make sure you are getting enough water. Your body will thank you!

- Eat organic
  - Support your local farmers. Go to the farmers markets near you and stock up on all the beautiful organic fruits and veggies. Your body, the farmers, and the planet will thank you!

- Be easy on yourself
  - Everyone makes mistakes. Don't be too hard on yourself, and pick yourself up when you fall. Go back to your WHY. You got this!

Remember these questions from Chapter 1? Use them as points to come back to. Hopefully by now, your answers are looking more like the answers below. I know that when I am more in health my answers are clearer and guide me towards health and vitality.

- Do you eat the same foods every day?
  - *No, I listen to my body and its needs. Most days I eat a salad OR a smoothie, but I have a variety of foods, and some days I have the cookie!*

- Are you food educated?
  - *Not only am I more educated about food now, I'm more educated about my body and its response to food as energy.*

- Do you read ingredient labels on packaged foods?
  - *Yes! I am looking for ingredients I know how to pronounce, and that my grandmother would recognize as food. I am looking for organic and non-GMO products that make me feel better and give me more energy and vitality. I understand this isn't always possible, like when I am on vacation, so I really try to do this as much as possible.*

- Do you think there is one way for you to eat?
  - *No. Every day is different. I listen to my body's needs. I pay attention to symptoms, so I know when to ease off of something. I know that I am constantly evolving.*

- Do you crave your favorite meals from your childhood and beyond?
  - *Yes, but I make them healthy now, and I make them differently based on my needs. I have different recipes that carry me to health (and now you have them too!). Sometimes I go*

for my favorite chocolate chip cookie, but if I need the sweet and reset I go for my cheat cookie dough balls that have very few ingredients. I can enjoy my mom's chili and the bread I learned to make in cooking school, all while feeling healthier than ever. We can have our cake, and eat it too!

- Do you care about conventional versus organic?
  - *Yes, because I understand that there is an industry out there that just wants to make money, and does not care about my health. I have to be responsible for my health, and that starts with making sure the foods I eat aren't sprayed with chemicals that we don't fully understand yet. Also, after learning that GMOs were added to the food supply in 1995, I definitely don't want my family or myself to be their experiment.*

Now that you are on the right path, what else can you do to help yourself, both body and mind? It's not just the food you take in that affects you.

- What media are you ingesting?
  - What are your sources?
  - Are you stuck on the negative in the news?

- What connections are you creating?
  - Do your relationships lift you up?
  - Do you feel better after being around your friends and family?

- What are you reading?
  - Do you read books that educate and uplift you?
  - Do you read books that bring you into fear and induce anxiety?

- What products (from cleaning to bathing) are you using in your life?
  - Do you know your senses take it all in through the mouth, eyes, nose, touch, and skin?
  - Are you ingesting toxins without realizing it?

I find that what I am feeding myself, in all areas of my life, is the one thing that makes the biggest difference. Look at what you are ingesting in all aspects of your life. When you know more, you fear less. Take the time to control the one thing you are able to—what you are feeding yourself. It all starts with an awareness of what you are bringing into your body.

I want you to start to have fun with food. Decide what lifestyle is best for you. After trying to incorporate more plants into your diet, try to find ways to keep it consistent. I hope I have shown you how eating more plant-based and organic can help guide you in your health. If you are anything like me and have realized the benefits of eating this way, then try to keep learning new recipes and trying out new products.

After many years of trying different things, I know that, for my body, I always feel my best if I have smoothies and salads on a regular basis, so if that makes you feel more healthful, I hope that these become new habits for you too.

Jumping off the yo-yo dieting train and eating plant-based gave me a whole new lease on life. I went from blah to fab, from dull to shiny. The beauty of it is that just incorporating more plant-based foods will help you too. It does not have to be a complete overhaul, but is based on daily steps and forming habits. I hope this has shown you that in so many ways YOU control your body's health with the food you eat.

Doesn't it feel good to feel good? Check in with yourself throughout this journey. Are there times where you stumble and maybe eat something that makes you feel less than spectacular? That's ok! Remember it for next time and know that if you ever stumble you can get it back. This is not an end-all-be-all, but a constant journey of striving to do better and learn what our bodies want and need.

Many clients I have worked with that continue to eat meat, do well with a 4-day 100% plant-based diet and 3 days with meat or dairy. This gives your body more time in an antioxidant state than in an immune response state. You also will be able to see what your body can take with animal products and if an over-abundance of them is causing your health problems. Remember that we are all different and you have to see what works for you. I wish I had a magic pill or shake I could give everyone that brought them into health, but it's for you to learn about yourself. I have plenty left to learn about myself and I find that often I get into patterns that don't work for me. Then I adjust. Do your best, try different things, and see what works for you.

I always say there are three types of vegans, ones for health, ones for animals, and ones for the planet. I fall under someone that is vegan for her health, but helping animals and the planet are a plus. There are a lot of things we can do better with. Animals and our planet should be at the top of our list. At least to live a little more naturally while we are here.

Small changes over time equal big changes. Being more plant-based means so much more to me than what I put on my plate. I do my best to walk my talk.

It only takes a little research to see that we can do better for ourselves. So that's what I did. I started making small changes in my life. I stopped using paper and plastic plates in my home and at parties. I began supporting restaurants that use biodegradable take out. I pack my own water bottle and, if I must splurge, I buy glass and reuse it. There are so many little things you can do. I just want you to start somewhere. Start exploring how you can reduce, reuse, and recycle in your life. Once I started, I began to see how things were made and if they didn't support my health or the planet's I would find a replacement or go without.

Changing the products we use, and reducing waste is so important for the planet. Don't forget, of all the things we can do for our health, and the health of our planet, cutting out meat is the biggest. I learned in the documentary *Cowspiracy* that if you replace your beef burger for a mushroom burger you would save more water than shortening your shower. You also contribute less carbon to the planet. And you are helping your body too.

Go back to the goals you created in Chapter 1. After reading this book do you feel that those goals are more attainable? I know from my experience, they are! Also, it's important to always be setting new goals, because we evolve as people, and want to be working toward new goals. If I kept the same goals I had throughout my life, I would be stuck in the same loop and never evolve. Our goals need to evolve when we are changing our lives for the better. I want to remind you to keep coming back to set goals for the body and health that you want.

Be a little easier on vegans, they are only trying to make the planet a better place. If you Google why people are vegan, you will see that there is so much room for improvement with everything when it comes to our food. I'm not here to shame you, but 90% of the meat at grocery stores and big box stores is factory farmed and the animals live in horrible conditions. The milk you drink harms the animals, so choose to get it from the smallest farms you can. If you need meat, frankly, who am I to tell you that you shouldn't have it. But instead of arguing with a vegan, maybe try to look at where you can be better.

Stumble with Grace

Look, it's not if, but when we will fall or stumble out of health and out of our goals. I still stumble all the time. I pivot very quickly these days though. I don't allow my health to get too far off track. I like feeling good. I hate feeling crappy. Still, I fall at times and I am learning to change those falls into stumbles.

It is so important to have intention for what you want to have in your life, for what you want to have your health and body look like. This is what you need to know so you can remember what you want when you start to get out of health. A goal is worth getting back on the horse for.

Ask yourself, what have I done for my body today?

Make a goal of committing to at least one thing. With everything our bodies do for us, what am I doing for my body? It is a symbiotic relationship.

Get real with yourself and see what isn't serving you in your life.

Make small changes. It starts with one step, one choice in the right direction to get back on track.

Make a promise to yourself to make YOU and your health a priority.

Remember you can always choose or find healthier versions of the foods you want to eat.

You are worth showing up for.

You made it! You're ready to take yourself on! You have decided your life can be better, healthier, and more fulfilling and you have taken that first precarious step. I am here to tell you that you can make it. You are powerful. You have the ability to shape your version of your dream life.

You can have the body, weight, self-honor, and life that you believe you deserve. When you take yourself on, change your habits, and live in intention, there is nothing out of your reach. All you have to do is be clear on what you want to create. My intention is to inspire you to soar by sharing what I have learned on my journey to health, so you can find yours. I want to guide you and hold space for you wherever you are and however far you want to go.

You have taken your first step, now let's take another. It's time for you to commit, because it's all about being present in life. It's all about the practice. It's all about the FOLLOW THROUGH! You must have an intention of why you want to divorce your diet and then put in the work. I have found no other way to take yourself on and get results. Whether in business, love, cleanses, or life in general, you need to be in it to win it. And you are!

It's official I grant you a divorce.

WELCOME to the rest of your wonderful new life!

XO,
Hollan

Now let's get you in the kitchen...
   Tools of the Trade

   Vitamix™ Blender—the best of the best in my opinion
   Cuisinart ood chopper (ranging from 2 to 11 cups)
   KitchenAid mixer
   Breville juicer
   Cuisinart blender stick
   Cutting board
   Sauté pans—stainless steel, various sizes
   Large boiling pot
   Pots and pans
   Cupcake pan
   Half sheet pan (cookie sheet)
   Glass baking dish 9" × 9"
   Glass baking dish 9" × 13"
   Strainer
   A good knife
   Bundt pan
   Can opener
   Ice cream maker
   Mixing spoons
   Skillet

APPENDIX

Chapter 1

Minor, Lloyd. "Why Medical Schools Need to Focus More on Nutrition." *School of Medicine*, Stanford University, 10 Oct. 2019, https://med.stanford.edu/school/leadership/dean/precision-health-in-the-news/why-medica-schools-need-focus-nutrition.html#:~:text=And%20a%20good%20place%20to,than%2020%20hours%20on%20nutrition.

Fox, Nick. "The Many Health Risks of Processed Foods." *LHSFNA*, Laborer's Health and Safety Fund of North America, 1 Feb. 2022, https://www.lhsfna.org/the-many-health-risks-of-processed-foods/.

Communications, Brigham and Women's Hospital. "Researchers Report Dramatic Rise in Cancer in People under 50." *Harvard Gazette*, Harvard Health Publishing, 9 Sept. 2022, news.harvard.edu/gazette/story/2022/09/researchers-report-dramatic-rise-inearly-onset-cancers/.

Chapter 2

What Happens to Your Food after You Eat It? - Gikids. North American Society for Pediatric Gastroenterology, Hepatology and Nutrition, https://www.gikids.org/files/documents/resources/Eat-E.pdf.

Ron. "The Game Changers - Revolutionary New Documentary about Meat, Protein, and Strength." *MindBody Medicine*, 1 Dec. 2019, https://www.healmindbody.com/do-you-want-to-improve-your-athletic-performance-and-feel-better/.

Lee, Janet. "Are Plant Proteins Complete Proteins?" *Consumer Reports*, Consumer Reports, 25 Feb. 2017, https://www.consumerreports.org/diet-nutrition/are-plant-proteins-complete-proteins/.

White, Dr. Ross. "7 Essential Nutrients Your Body Needs." *Wellness Daily*, Wellness Daily Australia, 4 June 2018, https://www.wellnessdaily.co.uk/health/7-essential-nutrients-your-body-needs.

Fields, Helen. "The Gut: Where Bacteria and Immune System Meet." *Johns Hopkins Medicine, John Hopkins Medicine*, Nov. 2015, https://www.hopkinsmedicine.org/research/advancements-in-research/fundamentals/in-depth/the-gut-where-bacteria-and-immune-system-meet.

"The Microbiome." *The Nutrition Source, 25 July 2022*, https://www.hsph.harvard.edu/nutritionsource/microbiome/.

Amos, Jennifer. "These Fish Have the Highest Level of Omega-3 Fatty Acids." *Tasting Table*, Tasting Table, 9 Sept. 2022, https://www.tastingtable.com/1000895/these-fishhave-the-highest-level-of-omega-3-fatty-acids/.

Group, Environmental Working. "Clean Fifteen™ Conventional Produce with the Least Pesticides." *EWG's 2022 Shopper's Guide to Pesticides in Produce | Clean Fifteen*, Environmental Working Group, 2022, https://www.ewg.org/foodnews/clean-fifteen.php.

Chapter 3

Campbell, T. Colin, and Thomas M. Campbell. *The China Study*. Macro, 2019.

Naftulin, Amanda MacMillan and Julia. "4 Science-Backed Health Benefits of Eating Organic." *Time*, Time, 27 July 2017, https://time.com/4871915/health-benefits-organic-food/.

"Organic for All." *Friends of the Earth*, 25 June 2021, https://foe.org/organic-for-all/.

Only organic. "Only Organic." *Only Organic*, https://www.onlyorganic.org/.

"Organic Food." *Encyclopædia Britannica*, Encyclopædia Britannica, Inc., https://www.britannica.com/topic/organic-food.

"GMO Facts - the Non-GMO Project." *The Non-GMO Project - Everyone Deserves an Informed Choice*, 2 Dec. 2022, https://www.nongmoproject.org/gmo-facts/.

Chapter 4

Neil-Sherwood, Dr. Michele. "The Power of the Sleep Cycle." *Functional Medical Institute*, 15 Nov. 2022, https://fmidr.com/the-power-of-the-sleep-cycle/.

Chapter 7

Starr, Michelle. "Your Body Makes 3.8 Million Cells Every
    Second. Most of Them Are Blood." *ScienceAlert*,
    23 Jan. 2021, https://www.sciencealert.com/
    your-body-makes-4-million-cells-a-second-and-most-of-
    them-are-blood.